STAYiNG ALiVE

Living Life with Longevity and Vitality

Dr. Vinny Leonti

Staying Alive: July 2022

ISBN: 978-1-64810-166-3

Printed in the United States of America

TABLE OF CONTENT

Acknowledgments & Dedications v

Preface vii

Introduction 1

Chapter 1 My Story. 3

Section I: Unwellness: What to do now. 19

Chapter 2 Where the World is Now 25

Chapter 3 Taking Stock: Where Are You Now? 33

Section II What you can do if you already have an issue 39

Chapter 4 Diet, Detox, & Supplements. 41

Chapter 5 Exercise and Activity. 85

Chapter 6 Sleep 91

Chapter 7 Stress Mitigation/Mental Emotional
Spiritual Health. 103

Chapter 8 Lifestyle. 111

Chapter 9 HBOT and Other Therapies. 117

Section III What Vitality and Vibrancy
can mean in our lives................................127

    Chapter 10 Contribution, Impact, Legacy.............131

Appendix A: Action Steps 139

Appendix B: Quick Start Guide 141

Appendix C: Explanations for the Quick Start Guide.......143

Biography 149

Index 151

References 155

ACKNOWLEDGMENTS & DEDICATIONS

To my Mom and Dad, who always made me feel loved and shaped who I am.

My wife, Sue Leonti, of almost 40 years, who has been with me through thick and thin. I could not have done it without her love, support and encouragement as we started and have grown Princeton Integrative Health and so much more!

My daughter Jenna Richardson, whose vision created Princeton Integrative Health and persuaded me to start a new career in Integrative Medicine. Her support has been invaluable through the years.

My son, Justin Leonti, MA, AMFT for his support and encouragement.

And for my grandchildren, Carter and Nyah, who inspire me to make the world a better place.

Dr. Sachin Patel who, through his Living Proof and Perfect Practice Mentorships, provided the support and guidance needed to kickstart our Integrative Medicine practice.

Dr. Tom Moorcroft who, through his Lyme Mentorship, helped me understand the complexities of Lyme Disease and other complex, chronic illness.

Sean Callagy, founder of Unblinded Sales Mastery, and everyone in Unblinded, for helping me to see that the world needed my vision and my message, now more than ever.

Dr. Jason Sonners, HBOT USA for his education about Hyperbaric Oxygen Therapy and support in bringing Hyperbaric Therapy to our community.

Lee Yonish, CNC for her important contributions to the Diet, Detox and Supplements chapter.

Michael Mras and Dr. Michelle Mras, for editing and bringing this book to life.

Dr. Ken Rochon 'Dr. Smiley', Founder of Perfect Publishing, and The KEEP SMILING Movement ☺, for believing in me and for his encouragement, his vision, and his indispensable help in completing this book and getting it published.

PREFACE

The greatest medicine of all is to teach people not to need it.
~Anonymous

Why did I write this book?

I wrote this book because I developed a life-threatening condition.

A life-threatening condition that I knew I was at risk for.

Avoiding this life-threatening condition encompassed my entire life, and was the core of my career.

I applied the latest conventional medical knowledge about risk, ate the American Heart Association recommended diet, and exercised regularly.

Despite all my efforts, I developed heart disease.

Fortunately, that was not the end of my journey.

Heart disease is where my journey begins.

I realized that the knowledge and insights I gained on that journey could save lives. I realized that it could save more lives than I saved during my entire 24-year career in Emergency Medicine.

How is that possible?

It is possible because I learned what truly matters in regard to our Health. I learned about the hidden risk factors that can be discovered with simple testing. When people learn about and implement these strategies, they will survive and they will thrive.

This is a book about my Life's Journey...

Ultimately, it is about all of us. How we can all change the trajectory of our life journey.

This is a book about Health, Joy, Vitality, Vibrancy and Hope.

Why did I write this book now?

I feel that we are at a Critical Crossroads in our Nation's history. I know that sounds melodramatic.

The news is rife with political divide, COVID mandates, and lifted mandates. The country is in turmoil.

But where there is turmoil, there is Hope. Hope for change, hope for a better way of doing things.

Hope for the Paradigm Shift.

COVID has wakened many people to the fact that our Conventional Medical System is lacking in many regards. This has been true for decades. Most people just weren't either aware or just did not want to think about it.

Why do I say we need a Paradigm Shift?

First, I recognized there is a problem. Let's take Heart Disease. It is still the number one killer for over 100 years running, It even outstrips COVID. It is the number one killer despite the Billions we spend on treating heart disease with Medications, Stents and other Procedures. The Annual Cost is $300 Billion. Yet, it is largely preventable.

With the current system of medications "a pill for an Ill", 7-minute doctor visits, the emphasis on treatment with procedures, it became apparent to me that the current system was failing to meet the needs of individual patients and the population as a whole.

My own journey with the Conventional Medical System, both as a patient and an insider, allowed me to understand how the system was failing. And my journey with Integrative Health, with its true partnership with patients and emphasis on prevention and regression of disease, showed me a new way that is as old as Hippocrates:

"Let food be thy medicine and medicine be thy food".

And an Ayurvedic Proverb:

"The importance of healthy food is exemplified by an Ayurvedic proverb: When the diet is wrong, medicine is of no use; when the diet is right, medicine is of no need".

(Warning: Do not stop your medications unless you are working with a doctor to make sure you can do so safely).

The insights I had directly led to my calling to educate people on how to lead their most Vibrant lives. They needed to know about their Hidden Risk Factors to avoid any premature threats to their Health and Vitality.

People need to know:

#1 The Conventional Medicine approach, with its overreliance on Medication and Procedures, puts some people's life at risk by not giving them a true picture of their health.

#2 True Health means not only to be free of disease, but to have the Vital, Vibrant Health that allows us to contribute to community, play with our grandkids, travel, ski or whatever it is your Heart and Soul desires.

I grew tired of all the death and disability I have seen from Cardiac disease, dementia, stroke, cancer, mental health which are all largely preventable.

I want to motivate people to take action.

If I can motivate people to take that first action step, then this book will be worth it. For initiating action often takes the greatest energy. Once action is initiated, it takes less effort to sustain it.

The sooner you make changes, the smaller the changes will need to be. Don't delay, putting this off for another day. Your changes, your effort in this arena, can literally be life-changing and life-saving. I know. I have seen the other side too often.

We can sum the book up as:

First Survive. Then Thrive. That's what I've learned to do. That's what I'm going to teach you.

There are others doing similar work. If you would like to read more, look up some of my favorites:

- Bradley Bale and Amy Doneen
  - Beat the Heart Attack Gene: The Revolutionary Plan to Prevent Heart Disease, Stroke, and Diabetes
  - Healthy Heart, Healthy Brain: The Personalized Path to Protect Your Memory, Prevent Heart Attacks and Strokes, and Avoid Chronic Illness
- Dale Bredesen
  - The End of Alzheimer's: The First Program to Prevent and Reverse Cognitive Decline
- Mimi Guarneri
  - The Heart Speaks: A Cardiologist Reveals the Secret Language of Healing
  - The Science of Natural Healing
  - 108 Pearls to Awaken Your Healing Potential: A Cardiologist Translates the Science of Health and Healing Into Practice
- Jack Wolfson
  - The Paleo Cardiologist: The Natural Way to Heart Health

- Mark Houston
  - Controlling High Blood Pressure through Nutrition, Supplements, Lifestyle and Drugs (with Lee Bell)
  - What Your Doctor May Not Tell You About Heart Disease

Who did I write this book for?

I wrote it for anyone not currently paying attention to their health

I wrote it for the Busy Account Executive

The Homemaker with Children

The Partier

People with lives so busy, they don't think they can find time to take care of their health.

For all, let me say, taking care of your health takes less time than you think.

And if you don't take the time to take care of your health, your health will take care of you.

INTRODUCTION

I could have died...died, like Jim Fixx , a physician who started the running movement, died in 1984 while out on a run. I was in shock when Dr. Jamar told me I had an 80% blockage in my LAD Coronary Artery, known as the Widowmaker, and they put a stent in. I could have died on that last run when I was seized by that crushing chest pain. Unstable Angina! I had been working to avoid this very fate my entire life. Without warning, I had developed Unstable Angina that could have killed me. Suddenly, feeling fragile, mortal and afraid, I questioned why this happened.

What had I done wrong???

This book will illustrate the lessons I learned on my health journey. It will teach you how to avoid what I suffered.

This book can be summed up as:

First Survive. Then Thrive. That's what I've learned to do. And that's what I'm going to teach you.

This book starts with my story and then is divided into 3 sections:

Section 1: Unwellness: What to do now

Section 2: Pivoting from Unwellness

Section 3: What Vitality and Vibrancy can mean in our lives

Finally, there is a Quick Start Guide as an appendix to get you started to better health.

Action Steps People Should Take Who Read This Book:

- Get Tested
- Eat Better
- Sleep Better
- Optimize Exercise and Activity
- Stress Management
- Mental, Emotional and Spiritual Health
- Improve Relationships
- Have the Energy, the Vitality to accomplish their goals and Legacy

This Book is meant to be literally a Life Changer.

CHAPTER 1

MY STORY

Fun Fact: At least 80% of heart attacks and Strokes are Preventable.[1] That should make people smile. ☺

June 14, 2012. Age 57. Wilson Regional Medical Center, Johnson City, NY

I was just coming out of anesthesia. I was still a little groggy. What was Doctor Jamar saying?

"It's a good thing you came in when you did. Your cardiac Cath showed that you have an 80% blockage in your left anterior descending coronary artery, and a 70% in the right coronary artery."

I thought maybe I misheard him.

"Excuse me. What did you say?"

Dr. Jamar said it a little more slowly this time so I would be able to grasp it.

"You have an 80% blockage in your Left Anterior Descending Artery and a 70% on your Right. We put in 2 stents."

I could not believe it. Left anterior descending artery, known as the widow maker. It's known as the widow maker because of its propensity to cause sudden death. Holy S#*t!!!

How could this happen to me? I was in shock. This could not be happening to me. Surprise, disbelief, grief all swirling around in my head and body.

I run marathons. I eat the American Heart Association (AHA) Diet. I never smoked. My cholesterol is normal. My Blood Pressure is normal.

I have none of the conventional Cardiac Risk factors and damn it, I run marathons! I run every day. I run to avoid heart disease. This is not right! How can this be? I couldn't grasp it.

"Dr. Jamar, how can this be? I run. I don't smoke. My cholesterol is average. I really don't have any risk factors."

"Your Dad. Your Family History of Heart Disease."

My Dad. My Dad who had a Heart Attack at the age of 47.

Sunday, February 9, 1969 Age 13. Valley Stream, NY

The Blizzard of 1969 in New York City wasn't supposed to be a blizzard at all. It was supposed to start as a snowfall and then change to rain later in the day. The blizzard did not follow that plan. Instead, temperatures plummeted, the wind howled and over a foot of snow was dumped on an unprepared city. People were out on the roads because there had been no warning to stay home. Thousands were stranded on the highway. Over 40 people died.

In Valley Stream, where I lived, closer to 2 feet of snow fell. I went outside to shovel the driveway with my Dad. That snow was heavy! My arms ached from that heavy, wet snow! Dad finally said it was time to go inside. What a relief!

What I did not realize was that Dad had developed crushing chest pain and was feeling lightheaded. He did not want to worry me or Mom, so he kept it to himself. He didn't want us to see he was feeling poorly, so he climbed that flight of steps upstairs (putting more strain on his heart) and laid down. He felt worse, started sweating profusely and realized something was terribly wrong. He later told me he suddenly realized he might die up there. He knew in his bones, and in his heart, he had to get downstairs. Mom took one look at his sweaty, grey face and called the Ambulance. I could not believe how bad my Dad looked. He had always seemed so strong and invincible. It was quite a shock and trauma to my 13-year-old self because that day I was terrified my Dad might die.

When the ambulance took him to the hospital in the middle of that storm, we were terribly worried. Would he be okay? Mom rode in the ambulance with him. I couldn't go to the hospital because of the storm. I continued to worry he might not make it.

Dad arrived at the hospital in bad shape. They called his doctor, but he couldn't make it in. Mom felt distraught and desperate. She felt Dad was going to die if he couldn't be evaluated by a doctor.

But then, at the hospital, was an amazing and caring Cardiologist, Dr. Sandhaus. He wasn't Dad's doctor. But after Mom spoke with him and pleaded for him to take a look at Dad, he consented. What a stroke of luck that turned out to be. He was amazing! He stayed at the hospital and monitored Dad closely. What a blessing! It was touch and go, but he brought Dad through. I had been so scared, but so relieved when Dad came home.

Dad's heart attack and recovery under Dr. Sandhaus care was a huge event at an impressionable time. I wanted to be a doctor like Dr. Sandhaus.

Many have those dreams of becoming a doctor, but not all succeed. I was lucky. I was blessed. I worked hard and loved to learn! I was a good student and never wavered. I got accepted to medical school early in my senior year of college. That was thrilling! I would soon be entering the hallowed halls of medicine. Able to help others.

As I progressed in my medical school training, I always took special note of the lessons on heart disease and prevention. Dad was a pack per day smoker. He was 60 lbs overweight. He did not do any regular physical activity. I was determined to avoid heart disease entirely. I would exercise. I would never smoke. I would check my cholesterol and blood sugar. I would eat the AHA diet. Do all the things Conventional Medicine said to do to prevent heart disease. I was determined to avoid the heart disease that had afflicted my Dad.

I took up running. I started my running career in medical school and capped it with my first marathon just before graduation.

I was running to avoid heart disease. Physically running from Heart Disease.

It appeared to be working. Dad had a Heart Attack at the age of 47. As I approached my 47th birthday, I had some trepidation, yet I sailed through that birthday without a hitch. My program was working, or so, I thought.

January 11,2011 Age 51 Hammond Hill State Forest, Freeville, NY

I loved Cross Country skiing. The freedom of being outside, the exertion of climbing hills, the thrill of the downhill runs. It was exhilarating for me. I got out whenever I could. But one day while I was out in the solitary backwoods of Hammond Hill, I had some Left-sided chest pain. Not a soul around. That realization was worrisome to me. I made it back without incident, but it left me feeling nervous. I decided to be evaluated. I had a Stress test and a CT Coronary Calcium score. Passed the stress test with no problem. I was in great shape. Coronary Calcium Score zero.

False alarm I thought. I'm all good.

June 11, 2012 Age 57 Apalachin, NY

Out for a routine run in the early morning. Days had been steamy with humidity, unusual for June. More like the dog days of August. At 6 AM, it was still comfortable. I'm cruising along with no issues. Then suddenly, out of nowhere, I develop a severe chest discomfort about a mile into a 3 mile run. I walk. Pain goes away. I run and pain returns. Huh, what is this, I wonder?

The Chinese food I had last night? Never made me feel this way before? I can't really wrap my head around what might be causing me to feel this way. I always complete my workouts. Today, I decided not to run the big hill. Sometimes the impact of the little decisions we make don't become apparent until later. Knowing what I know now, I know that decision saved my life. It gives me chills when I think how that day could have ended so differently.

I made it back to my car without incident. I told my wife and promised I would call a Cardiologist. Two days later, I'm having a stress test. I'm cruising along, barely out of breath, when I hear the Cardiologist order the test stopped. I look at the cardiac monitor and realize my ST segments are depressed, a sign of ischemia, meaning there is a blockage and not enough blood is getting to a segment of the heart. Then they do an Echocardiogram to look at how the heart muscle is beating. When there is ischemia, heart muscle function should be depressed. The Echocardiogram is normal. Conflicting information. I hold out the hope to myself that perhaps that ST segment depression was a false positive, that I didn't really have ischemia.

I decide to go through with the Cardiac catheterization (cath) anyway. I secretly think it will be fine.

Thursday is the day of the cath. I am told if they find blockages and have to put in stents, I will have to spend the night. If no stents, then I can go home. I do not cancel work the next day thinking I will be going home.

Needless to say, I did not make it to work the next day. This was the cath that showed my blockage of the Widowmaker and the Right Coronary Artery.

I am not a person prone to depression. I am usually upbeat, seeing the silver lining in every cloudy situation. But this felt different. I was overcome with emotion. There was depression, grief, and a feeling of loss. I felt disoriented. It was as if everything I had studied and learned to avoid heart disease was incomplete or wrong. It gave me that feeling you get when you are certain, certain something is true, and you find that it is not. That sick feeling in the pit of your stomach. Your whole world is rocked.

If I could not avoid heart disease with its risk of sudden death, then what chance did non-medical people have? I was disconcerted. I didn't know what to do.

After going through this phase, I decided I needed to do everything in my power to find the truth, in order to understand how this could happen. If I couldn't understand, how could I avoid this happening again? How could I really help others? I started asking questions of the cardiologists, and my primary care physician. How did this happen? Why did this happen to me? The only answer I got was, "Your Family History?" What? That's it? I can't change that. Is your Family History truly your destiny? I did not want to believe that. No one could give me a satisfactory explanation. No one could say what in my Family History had led to my coronary blockages.

I became disillusioned with Conventional Medicine. When my daughter Jenna became an Integrative and Functional Diagnostic Nutritionist, she shared what she was learning. I saw that there was a more Integrative and Holistic way. I learned how the low fat, high carb AHA Diet, which was far from preventing Heart Disease, had contributed to a multi-generational cycle of obesity, Insulin Resistance and Diabetes. Which all raised the risk of Heart Disease. I started to learn how my nutrition and stressful Emergency Room work life had played a role in my heart disease. I started to see that Family History is not your destiny. I was learning that the choices we make, our lifestyle, is more important than our Family History. This is such a powerful and inspiring outlook!

June 2016 to January 2017. Age 62. Lawrenceville, NJ

When Jenna, my daughter, proposed we could start an Integrative, Holistic Medical Practice in Lawrenceville, NJ, I was skeptical. I had lived in NY all my life. My wife, Sue, and I would have to uproot our entire lives and essentially start over at the age of 62. I was getting ready to retire. Just a few more years. Didn't she know that? Apparently, she heard, but she was not dissuaded. She kept talking with me, telling me how we would have much more power and control to help people if we created this practice. She is very persuasive. She helped me overcome my doubts and fears. Finally, I agreed and Princeton Integrative Health opened its doors in January 2017.

My Heart Health journey was still incomplete. I felt I had some answers, but not enough of a picture to be satisfied. I found Dr. Chip Whitney, a Family Medicine trained Integrative Physician, in Washington Crossing, PA. One of his specialties is Heart Attack and Stroke Prevention. Working with him, I uncovered my undiagnosed Risk factors. I call these the Hidden Risk factors.

What were my Hidden Risk Factors? Turns out I had an inherited Lipoprotein disorder, an elevated Lipoprotein-a (Lp-a). Lp-a is a risk factor present in 20% of the population, often a culprit in premature heart disease of healthy people in their 40s or younger. Lp-a is not tested for on standard blood tests.

ApoE is a gene with 3 variations named ApoE 2, ApoE 3, or ApoE 4. You inherit one gene from each parent so you can be a 2/2, 3/3, 4/4 or 2/4, 3/4, etc. The importance of this is that ApoE 2 or 3 don't confer any increased risk of heart disease, but ApoE 4 is a very inflammatory genotype and confers at least a 50% increased risk of heart disease and dementia. I am a 4/4, the most inflammatory genotype.

I also had high risk bacteria in my mouth, bacteria known to contribute to inflammation in the arteries. I had this despite going to the dentist every 6 months for cleanings. I now had a clearer understanding of my Hidden Risk factors and answers to the questions that plagued me.

These insights directly led to my calling to educate people how to lead their most Vibrant lives. They needed to know about their Hidden Risk Factors to avoid any premature threats to their Health and Vitality.

People need to know:

#1 the Conventional Medicine approach, with its overreliance on Medication and Procedures, puts some people's life at risk by not giving them a true picture of their health.

#2 True Health means not only to be free of disease, but to have the Vital, Vibrant Health that allows us to contribute to community, play with our grandkids, travel, ski or whatever it is your Heart and Soul desires.

March 2020 to March 2022 Ages 64 to 66 Lawrenceville, NJ

COVID. Such an unsettling time to test our precepts.

In order for us to keep our practice viable, we had to adjust. People were scared, huddled in their homes. We went heavily into telemedicine. This turned out to be life-saving for all involved.

We were able to meet the challenges of our practice and also the challenges many families faced. My wife and I were needed to help care for our grandchildren, Nyah, age 2 and Carter, age 6, when COVID started. I am so thankful that, by following the principles of health that we espouse, that we have the vitality and energy needed to meet one of the most demanding and challenging (but rewarding) situations that I have ever encountered... grandchildren.

We also met the challenges COVID posed to our own personal health. Having Heart Disease is known to raise the risk of severe illness or death from COVID. That was scary. We took our precautions, but being in health care, there is a certain amount of risk. I was put to the test in November 2021 when I contracted COVID. But, despite my apprehension, my case was mild with body aches for 4 days and fatigue for 12. My Program worked as well as could be hoped!

How does this story end?

That ending continues to be written. What I can tell you is this:

I feel as vibrant and alive now as I ever have. I have started a journey to save people's lives and to change healthcare in America for the better. On this journey, I have met amazing people who have helped me on my way.

I know this would not have happened had I not chosen this path, which has led to mission and purpose, energy and vitality, smiles and laughter all while spearheading a deadly serious purpose.

So please, hear what I have to say. It could save your life.

My primal Heartache was seeing my Dad suffer his heart attack and eventually die from heart disease; further Heartache when I developed heart disease and then my older brother was also diagnosed. All the males in our nuclear family. This was frightening, but learning the true causes of this so I may help others has been the joy of my life. You need to take action! Action to assess your own Heart Health.

This is how I turn Heartache into Hope.

Why do I do this?

I feel driven to do this for a few reasons. First, my own Family History and personal experience, the trauma of seeing my dad nearly die, the shock and trauma of developing my own heart disease, and then my brother. All the males in my family afflicted. Yet we did not smoke. I knew there had to be a better way to assess risk. Once I found that, I knew I had to give back to my community and to the world. I had seen so much sudden death in my time as an ER Doctor. I am impassioned to change that pattern, to prevent the heartache, tragedy and trauma that happens when someone dies unexpectedly before their time.

In my practice, I was quietly helping one person at a time. Then 2 things occurred that made me decide that I needed to raise awareness, to help not only those who came to my practice, but people I might never meet.

I joined a Mentorship called Unblinded. Unblinded helps people to see what they need to take their business to the next level. During a weekend retreat with the group, Sean Callagy, the Founder, was having pointed conversations with people in front of the group. Loving Interventions and Confrontations about what was holding them back. My turn came. I hate being in front of a group like this. He asked if I was making the contacts I needed to raise awareness and grow my business. I hated putting myself out to people like that. I told him I was not.

Sean: Can your knowledge and skills help people become healthier?

Me: Of course

Sean: Can it potentially save their lives?

Me: Yes.

Sean: And you are not reaching out to people to tell them that?

Me: No

Sean: Why are you holding back and not telling people that? What are you afraid of? Are you afraid of being rejected?

Me: Yes

Sean: And you're going to let that fear hold you back? Do you realize how selfish that is?

And in that moment, it hit me. I was being selfish by trying to protect myself. I needed to play a bigger game, to really put myself out there. How else was I going to change the world of Medicine, change the way that game is played?

I needed to become part of shifting the Medical Paradigm.

For more info on Unblinded, go to:
  https://unblindedmastery.com/

The second thing that happened was in the category of doing something that does not seem significant in the moment, but has a huge impact in your life. I serendipitously gave a ride to Dr. Ken Rochon, Dr. Smiley and to Dr. Andrea Adams-Miller. Unblinded was helping the American Foundation for the Blind fundraise for its 100th Anniversary. It was decided that there would be a major fundraiser with celebrities and NFL and MLB stars to help raise money. They decided they would open Helen Keller's Time Capsule to bring an even more special allure to the event. Tickets were going for $1000 apiece, but it seemed too special an event to pass up.

I was looking forward to the event. I had my black tie and 3-piece suit ready. This was going to be a big deal. They were bringing in professional photographers to record the Gala. The photographers were flying into Philadelphia, coming to Princeton to their hotel but needed a ride to NY. When I heard about their request, I offered to give them a ride. I lived 10 minutes from Princeton, so it was not a big deal. I did not know them personally, but knew they were with Unblinded, so I wanted to help out. Just the common courtesy and help we all give without thinking much about it.

There was terrible weather that day, severe thunderstorms with lightning and hail. Their plane had to land in DC and sat on the tarmac for 4 hours. By the time they were able to get to Philly and then Princeton, we would be over an hour late to the Gala. Ken and Andrea called and asked what I wanted to do. They would completely understand if I did not want to wait and miss the first hour of the Gala, they could call an Uber, etc., etc. I knew the quickest way they would get to NYC was if I waited and took them. So I did.

The drive was grueling. Along with the lightning, there was a heavy, drenching, open firehose type of rain, with no let-up the entire 90-minute drive. Visibility was poor and the traffic was moving, but heavy. Ken was sitting up front with me and we started having conversation about what we did in life. I told him I was an Integrative Physician and we talked about that. He told me he was a publisher, an author and had co-founded the Keep Smiling movement. He told me he likes to help people write and publish their books. He had helped his son Kenny (K3) Rochon III, write his first book, "Kenny's Favorite Jokes". Kenny was selling it on Amazon and earning commissions!

Hmmm…I had always thought I should write a book. Many people in the Integrative Medicine space write books. I really wanted to write a book and get my message out into the world. If Ken could help his 7-year-old write a book, maybe he could help me?!?

I half-jokingly asked Ken, "So when are you going to help me write my book?" Ken responded, "What do you want to write about?" A discussion of my ideas followed for the rest of the ride. Even with the terrible weather, the time flowed by and we got to Tribeca Rooftop where the Gala was being held. I dropped them at the door and drove around looking for a place to park.

The Gala was a smashing success. Ken and Andrea took great pictures. Finally, the time for the much-anticipated opening of Helen Keller's 1934 time capsule arrived. There was a picture of Helen Keller; a congratulatory letter from President Franklin D. Roosevelt; and a broadcast of the original Time capsule ceremony originally broadcast by NBC, amongst other items.[2] Discussing the contents was absorbing and interesting. It was over all too soon and we got back in the car for the ride back.

Our conversation about my book resumed where we left off. Ken said, "Dr. Vinny, for waiting for us, being willing to miss the first hour of the Gala, for the kindness you have shown us, I will help you publish your book. No matter how long it takes." Ken was true to his word. And the rest, as they say, is about to become history.

For more info on Dr. Ken Rochon and Umbrella Syndicate, go to:
https://www.TheUmbrellaSyndicate.com
https://www.facebook.com/TheUmbrellaSyndicate/

For more information about the Keep Smiling Movement, go to:
https://thekeepsmilingmovement.com/
https://www.facebook.com/KeepSmilingMovement/

For more information about Amplifluence, go to:
https://amplifluence.com
https://www.facebook.com/groups/619796712385348

SECTION I:

UNWELLNESS: WHAT TO DO NOW

An Ounce of Prevention is worth a Pound of Cure.
~Benjamin Franklin

The secret to living well and longer is: eat half, walk double, laugh triple and love without measure.
~Tibetan Proverb

The New Medical Paradigm

Taking Stock: Where are we at this point in time. COVID has made clear what has been apparent to many for a long time.

The American Health Care System has been failing to provide good health for Americans. It has pivoted from quality care to quantity care. No longer do doctors have the time to sit down and get to know their patients and their unique medical histories. This is critical to the understanding of inherent issues and ensuring the proper treatment is prescribed and followed.

The end result is "Cookie Cutter" medicine. What I mean by this is the use of "if/then" statements. "Do you eat right?" If not, tell them to eat right. "Do you exercise enough?" If not, tell them to work out more. You get the point. This also manifests in other areas like weight. When you go into the doctor's office, they take your height and weight. Those two facts, coupled with your gender, give them an "approximate BMI". That number does not take into account for physique. For example, bodybuilders will always rate "obese" using only these three factors.

This goes toward medications as well. If a test has an abnormal result, prescribe medicine A. If that does not work, prescribe medicine B. What this does not take into account is the patient history. Namely, why are the test results abnormal? What is the patient doing or not doing that could cause the abnormalities? To modern medicine, it is quicker and easier to medicate than to change lifestyles.

According to an industry insider, the biggest problems with The U.S. HealthCare System:[3]

- High Costs of Care
- Lack of Insurance Coverage
- Lack of Transparency
- Difficulty in finding physicians and specialists
- The growing concerns about specialists' burnout are also rising.

Another article by a Harvard Doctor and Senior Faculty Editor raises similar issues:[4]

- The cost is enormous
  - High cost, not highest quality
  - Financial Burden
- Access is uneven
  - Health insurance is tied to employment
  - Healthcare disparities
  - Health insurers may discourage care to hold down costs
- Investments in healthcare seem misdirected
  - Emphasizing technology and specialty care (rather than preventative care)
  - Overemphasizing procedures and drugs
  - Stifling innovation
  - Fragmented care
  - Defensive medicine (offered primarily to minimize lawsuits)

The modern medical system is a great system for acute care. If you break a bone, you develop an infection, hard to beat conventional medical care.

If you have a complex, chronic illness, it's overreliance on medications and procedures prevents true health and health care from occurring.

Type 2 Diabetes

Let's take a look at Type 2 diabetes. Type 2 diabetes is not a problem of lack of Insulin. That's Type 1 Diabetes. Type 2 diabetes is characterized by high Insulin, Insulin Resistance and elevated blood sugars

Type 2 Diabetes has been increasing in this country for the last three decades, year after year.[5]

Are there no new diabetes medications to deal with this growing problem?

Of course there are. New medications are approved all the time.

QUESTION: If medications and insulin were the answer to Type 2 diabetes, would it still be in the top 10 (#7) of leading causes of death?[6] Individuals with diabetes have a twofold to threefold increased risk of mortality compared to individuals without diabetes.[7]

Answer: I think you know the answer. If medications and Insulin were the answer, death rates would be lower.

How do we affect this problem? Let's take a look at another example before we answer that question.

Heart Disease

Coronary Artery Disease, at its Heart, is a disease of Inflammation. It is a disease of Inflammation driven by what we eat, our lifestyle behaviors and other modifiable risk factors. We will delve into this more deeply in this book.

An estimated 80% of cardiovascular disease, including heart disease and stroke, is preventable.[8]

The Cleveland Clinic feels "90 Percent of Heart Disease is Preventable through Healthier Diet, Regular Exercise, and Not Smoking."[9]

But, as my story illustrates, while the focus on diet, exercise and smoking in the general population will lower heart disease dramatically, it is not enough. The new medical paradigm will look at each individual's risk factors, including what I call the Hidden Risk factors not routinely tested for. This allows the creation of a personalized, precision plan for each individual, much more powerful than focusing on the general, population based, one size fits all of conventional medicine.

Bottom line, medicine focused on individual history, family history and holistically on five key areas will have better, longer lasting, and more personal results:

- Diet
- Exercise
- Sleep
- Mental Health
- Lifestyle

These are the areas we will go over in detail in section II of this book.

CHAPTER 2

WHERE THE WORLD IS NOW

The good physician treats the disease; the great physician treats the patient who has the disease.
~William Osler, Father of Modern Medicine

Until we understand the problem, we can't start to look at how to fix it. Let's start with an assessment of where the world is now, health-wise. Just a warning, this section may have content disturbing to some viewers, because it's a pretty bleak view of the state of health in America.

Each year, the American Heart Association (AHA), in conjunction with the National Institutes of Health and other government agencies, brings together in a single document the most up-to-date statistics related to heart disease, stroke, and cardiovascular risk factors.[10]

- **Cardiovascular Health**- 70% of Cardiovascular deaths (CVD) were attributed to people with poor cardiovascular health. If everyone had high cardiovascular health, it is estimated that we could prevent 2 million deaths per year. Even if we could get people to moderate cardiovascular health, it is estimated it could prevent 1.2 million deaths per year.
- **Smoking/Tobacco Use**- Although cigarette smoking has been declining for the last 20 years, it is still the leading cause of preventable disease and death in the United States.[11]
  - Cigarette smoking kills more than 480,000 Americans each year
  - The United States spends more than $300 billion a year on smoking-related illness, including more than $225 billion in direct medical care for adults and $156 billion in lost productivity
- **Physical Activity and Sedentary Behavior**- Only 54% of people get enough exercise. Adults (sixty and over) who are physically active are at a reduced risk for:
  - CVD mortality (25%–40% risk reduction)
  - All-cause mortality (22%–35%)
  - Breast cancer (12%–17%)
  - Prostate cancer (9%–10%)
  - Depression (17%–31%)

All while experiencing better quality of life, healthier aging trajectories, and improved cognitive functioning.

- **Nutrition**- Eating 5 (vs 2) servings of fruits and vegetables daily was associated with:
  - 13% lower total mortality
  - 12% lower CVD mortality

- ○ 10% lower cancer mortality
- ○ 35% lower respiratory disease mortality
- **Overweight and Obesity**- The prevalence of obesity is increasing rapidly.
  - ○ Males increased from 27.5% to 43.0% and severe obesity increased from 3.1% to 6.9%.
  - ○ Females increased from 33.4% to 41.9% and severe obesity from 6.2% to 11.5%.
- **High Blood Cholesterol and Other Lipids**- In 2015 to 2018, total cholesterol ≥200 mg/dL was present in 38.1% of adults, low-density lipoprotein cholesterol ≥130 mg/dL was present in 27.8% of adults, triglycerides ≥150 mg/dL were present in 21.1% of adults, high-density lipoprotein cholesterol <40 mg/dL was present in 17.2% of adults.
- **High Blood Pressure**- From 2009 to 2019, the death rate attributable to high BP increased 34.2%, and the actual number of deaths attributable to high BP rose 65.3%.
- **Diabetes**- In 2015-2018, an estimated 28.2 million adults (10.4%) had diagnosed diabetes, 9.8 million adults (3.8%) had undiagnosed diabetes, and 113.6 million adults (45.8%) had pre-diabetes.
- **Kidney Disease**- Overall prevalence of chronic kidney disease (estimated glomerular filtration rate <60 mL·min−1·1.73 m−2 or albumin-to-creatinine ratio ≥30 mg/g) was 14.9% (2015–2018). Medicare spent $81 billion caring for people with chronic kidney disease and $49.2 billion on those with end-stage renal disease in 2018.
- **Sleep**- Overall, 65.2% met the recommended sleep duration of ≥7 hours.
  - ○ 11.8% of people reported a sleep duration ≤5 hours,
  - ○ 23.0% reported 6 hours
  - ○ 29.5% reported 7 hours

- 27.7% reported 8 hours
- 4.4% reported 9 hours
- 3.6% reported ≥10 hours
- **Total Cardiovascular disease**- In 2020, roughly 19 million deaths were attributed to cardiovascular disease globally (an 18.7% increase from 2010).
- **Stroke**- Some good news, incidences of stroke are declining.
- **Brain Health**- Alzheimer disease and related dementia was the fourth most prevalent neurological disorder in the United States (2.9 million people). Among neurological disorders, Alzheimer disease and related dementia was the leading cause of mortality in the United States ahead of stroke.
- **Quality of Care**- Compared with 2019, a lower proportion of sudden death cases received bystander cardiopulmonary resuscitation in 2020, and use of automated external defibrillators was lower. There were also longer emergency medical services response times and lower survival to hospital discharge. Those are likely related to the COVID-19 pandemic.

With that in mind, let's look at the Leading Causes of Death in the United States. Notice the addition of COVID-19 which entered the chart at number three.

Leading Causes of Death (with numbers) in the United States (2020)[12]
- Heart disease: 696,962
- Cancer: 602,350
- COVID-19: 350,831
- Accidents (unintentional injuries): 200,955

- Stroke (cerebrovascular diseases): 160,264
- Chronic lower respiratory diseases: 152,657
- Alzheimer's disease: 134,242
- Diabetes: 102,188
- Influenza and pneumonia: 53,544
- Nephritis, nephrotic syndrome, and nephrosis: 52,547

So, where can we start? Let's looks at what we can do to change the numbers. In some studies, up to half of all premature deaths in the U.S. could be prevented through modifiable habits, the CDC puts that number lower, at 20% to 40%.[13] Unfortunately, while there has been progress in reducing early deaths in the United States from certain causes (i.e., tobacco and alcohol use) those are offset by increases in deaths linked to other factors, (i.e., poor diet and lack of physical activity). [14]

Leading Preventable Causes of Death[15][16]
1. Cigarettes
2. Obesity
3. Alcohol

Heart Disease and Stroke

Nearly 1 in 3 deaths in the US each year is caused by heart disease and stroke. At least 200,000 of these deaths could have been prevented through changes in health habits, such as stopping smoking, more physical activity, and less salt in the diet; and managing high blood pressure, high cholesterol, and diabetes.[17]

Dementia

Studies show that healthy behaviors, which can prevent some kinds of cancer, type 2 diabetes, and heart disease may also reduce your risk for cognitive decline. Although age, genetics, and family history can't be changed, the Lancet Commission on dementia prevention, intervention, and care suggests that addressing risk factors may prevent or delay up to 40% of dementia cases.[18]

Here's what you can do:

- Quit smoking. Quitting smoking may help maintain brain health and can reduce your risk of heart disease, cancer, lung disease, and other smoking-related illnesses.
- Maintain a healthy blood pressure level.
- Be physically active. CDC studies show physical activity can improve thinking, reduce risk of depression and anxiety and help you sleep better.
- Maintain a healthy weight. Establish and maintain a lifestyle including healthy eating and regular exercise.
- Get enough sleep. A third of American adults report that they usually get less sleep than seven hours a night.
- Stay engaged. Get involved in your community.
- Manage blood sugar. Especially if you have diabetes.

Cancer[19]

Cancer is the second leading cause of death in the United States, but many kinds of cancer (e.g., breast, cervical, and colorectal) can be prevented or caught early through screening. Other kinds can be prevented—for example, cervical cancer through vaccination and colorectal cancer through removal of abnormal growths in the colon and rectum before they turn into cancer.

Leading risk factors for preventable cancers are:
- Smoking
- Too much UV radiation (from the sun or tanning beds)
- Being overweight or having obesity
- Drinking too much alcohol

CHAPTER 3

TAKING STOCK: WHERE ARE YOU NOW?

How do I do this?

To effectively prevent heart disease, you must assess the conventional risk factors (e.g., smoking, cholesterol, etc.) as well as take an in-depth look at Inflammation, Insulin Resistance, Sleep apnea, and assessing inherited risk factors. You can get a specialized Vascular Ultrasound (a CIMT) to assess the health, inflammation and plaque in your arteries. This will let you and your doctor know how aggressively we need to intervene.

I do this by listening to each person, finding out what's important to them, and helping them to reach their goals.

I recommend everyone assess:

Your eating habits:

Sugar and carb content

Organic or not

Activity: 25-30 minutes of moderate activity per day

Sleep: 6 hours is the bare minimum, 7 hours or more is the CDC recommendation

Stress and Mental Health: How are you coping, my friend?

Find a doctor who can help you assess your health.

You will have to find a doctor who can help you identify your Hidden Risk factors. To do this, you have to get tests not normally performed in routine testing. It's imperative to identify the factors in your family history like those that caused my blockage and nearly killed me and have killed countless others.

A thorough history and physical to include bloodwork identifying:

- Lipid profile with particle numbers
- Lipoprotein-a
- Genetic markers
- Inflammatory markers
- Blood sugar and Insulin Resistance Markers
- Thyroid testing
- Hormones

Sleep Apnea Testing—a massively underdiagnosed cause of Heart problems, high blood pressure and dementia.

Oral Health and Oral Microbiome Testing—Bacteria from the Oral Microbiome have been implicated in blood vessel and brain inflammation leading to heart attack and dementia.

EKG—Looks at the electrical activity of the heart. Good to have as a baseline so changes can be more easily detected. It can also be done in conjunction with a stress test (i.e., treadmill) to make your heart work progressively harder to help identify blockages.

CIMT: Carotid Intima Media Thickness Ultrasound. A specialized Vascular Ultrasound that tells us the state of health of your Arteries.

These tests can predict who is at risk for Vascular Events such as heart attack and stroke years, even decades, before the events. This allows people to change their diet and lifestyle behaviors to prevent heart attack and stroke.

These tests will provide you a baseline of where you are currently and a roadmap for improving your health.

COVID

Although restrictions are being lifted as infections and deaths from COVID-19 continue to decrease, the United States recently surpassed a somber milestone—one million deaths.[20] COVID is not done and there is always the possibility that another stronger variant will emerge. As such, I want to include guidance to better protect you from getting COVID as well as what to do if you do catch it.

How to protect yourself and your family from COVID-19, based on the video by Dr. David Price, a Critical Care Doctor at Weill-Cornell Medical Center. Dr. Price is at the epicenter of this pandemic in the US. His observations are based on seeing actual patients and seeing how they are getting infected. His observations give hope to all of us.

His video can be found on-line:
https://vimeo.com/399733860?fbclid=IwAR2a7p-qZ5_k1Gn-0yogIedJUBLRdBQotA3XIZuGlR3elheHDUrehHqHHJFc

In summary, follow these rules and you are unlikely to get COVID-19 and we can protect ourselves and our families:

1. **Constantly wash or Sanitize (alcohol based) your hands.** If you touch anything that anyone else has touched: door handles, elevator buttons, packages: just wash or sanitize your hands afterward. If you are taking care of someone with COVID-19, make sure you wash your hands.
2. **Constantly work on avoiding connection between your hand and face**
3. **Wear a mask** or even a bandana or scarf to help with training ourselves on breaking the hand face connection.
4. **Maintain Social Distance of 3 to 6 feet.** If you can do this, your chances of contracting COVID-19 drop toward Zero even if you are out in public for a walk, exercising, etc. This makes sense as we know it spreads through saliva droplets which can only travel a limited distance and not aerosol (unless you are doing medical procedures) which can travel much further.

Those are the simple rules to protect us and our loved ones.

Dr. Price goes into much more detail. I shared his video on my Facebook page so you can watch it and get the information.[21] Please share with your families, loved ones and associations. It may feel daunting, but this -1-hour video is worth it.[22]

Supplements to prevent and manage Coronavirus.

NOTE: If you are having severe symptoms, please go to the Hospital.

2 Key Questions:

1. How best to support immunity to avoid infection?
2. How best to support people who get infected to make the clinical course as mild as possible?

First, supporting the body's ability to fight infection equals prevention. Prevention in the sense that your Immune System will be in an optimal state. This is for everyone who has not been infected. The first step is to optimize lifestyle: sleep well, reduce stress, decrease sugar and carbs, eat high potassium foods, and an anti-inflammatory, phytonutrient rich diet.

Foundational Supplements

- Vitamin D 5000 - 10,000IU daily (check level if taking 10,000 IU daily for more than 2 months)
- Vitamin A 5000 – 10,000IU daily
- Vitamin E 200 – 400mg daily
- Vitamin C 1gm daily

- Melatonin 5mg daily
- Quercetin 250mg 2 times/day
- NAC 600mg 2 times/day
- Reishi Mushroom Spores or coffee – Organo is the brand we use
- Curcumin 500mg 2 times/day
- (High Risk patients should also take Glutathione 500mg up to 4 times daily)
- TH1 Support for those with the highest risk. TH1 are Immune Cells that help strengthen and balance the Immune System

Second, how best to support someone infected is to essentially ramp up the Foundational Support Supplements. If someone's inflammation appears to be getting out of control, additional anti-inflammatory support is needed. These steps would have to be done under the guidance of a professional.

SECTION II:

WHAT YOU CAN DO IF YOU ALREADY HAVE AN ISSUE

You never know how strong you are,
until being strong is the only choice you have
~Bob Marley

So what if you've had an event or told you are at risk, what then?

You're scared or confused, what do you do now?

In this section, we are going to look at your diet, exercise, sleep, mental health, and lifestyle. Understand that these are all closely interrelated. You can't ignore one or two categories and expect positive results across the board. At the same time, positive effects do bleed over. For example, working out will help your weight, your mental health and your sleep.

CHAPTER 4
DIET, DETOX, & SUPPLEMENTS

What we eat and drink (and think too) becomes the matrix of our cells, tissues, organs, and body.
~Lee Yonish[23]

The natural healing force within each one of us is the greatest force in getting well. Our food should be our medicine. Our medicine should be our food.
~Hippocrates

What you eat has a huge impact on your health. As society moves forward, our food supply is less fresh, is reliant on fewer and fewer crops that have been sprayed with chemicals, more processed and more additives (steroids, antibiotics, preservatives, dyes, etc.). In other words, we are not eating close to nature, even though our genes and biology require us to do so.

That said, despite enormous advances in science and medicine, it is no surprise that obesity continues to be a problem worldwide. We are metabolically hampered by our modern lifestyle and industrial food supply. Many chronic diseases (e.g., diabetes, hypertension, and heart disease) are closely tied to obesity, and all are byproducts of our poor diets and lifestyle.[24]

There is no shortage of recommendations coming from various private and public entities. For example, the American Heart Association has published guidelines concerning diet and lifestyle recommendations for preventing and managing cardiovascular disease.[25] The AHA says:

Burn what you consume

- Food labels are normally based on a 2000 calorie per day diet. This will vary on many factors including age, gender and level of physical activity.
- If you want to lose weight, eat fewer calories or increase the amount of calories you burn through physical activity.

Physical Activity

- You should aim for 150 minutes of moderate physical actively or 75 minutes of vigorous physical active per week.
- Spread your workouts throughout the week.
- Take every opportunity to get some exercise (e.g., stairs vs elevator, park further away, walk to someone's desk rather than call or e-mail.

Eat an overall healthy dietary pattern that emphasizes:

- Fruits and vegetables
- Whole grains
- Healthy sources of protein (mostly plants such as legumes and nuts; fish and seafood; low-fat or nonfat dairy; and, if you eat meat and poultry, ensuring it is lean and unprocessed)
- Liquid non-tropical vegetable oils
- Minimally processed foods
- Minimized intake of added sugars
- Foods prepared with little or no salt
- Limit or avoid alcohol intake

These standards apply whether you eat at home or out. Look for the Heart-Check mark to find foods that have been certified by the American Heart Association as heart-healthy.

Our federal government also has a set of recommendations:

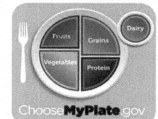

Fruits:
Focus on fruits.
- Eat a variety of fruit.
- Chose fresh, frozen, canned or dried fruit.
- Go easy on fruit juices.

Vegetables:
Vary your veggies.
- Eat more green dark veggies.
- Eat more orange veggies.
- Eat more dry beans and peas.

Physical Activity
Find your balance between food & physical activity.
- Be physically active for 30 minutes most days of the week.
- Children and teenagers should be physically active for 60 minutes everyday or most days of the week.

Oils:
Know your fats.
- Make most of your fat sources from fish, nuts and vegetable oils.
- Limit solid fats like butter, stick margarine, shortening, and lard.

Milk:
Get your calcium-rich foods.
- Go low-fat or fat-free
- If you don't or can't consume milk, chose lactose-free products or other calcium sources.

Grains:
Make at least half your grains whole.
- Eat at least 3 ounces of whole grain bread, cereal, rice, or pasta everyday.
- Look for the word "whole" before the grain name on the list of ingredients.

Meats & Beans
Go lean on protein.
- Choose low-fat or lean meats and poultry.
- Bake it, broil it or grill it.
- Vary your choices with more fish, beans, peas, nuts, and seeds.

Source: ChooseMyPlate.gov[26]

MyPlate is the current nutrition guide published by the USDA Center for Nutrition Policy and Promotion, a food circle depicting a place setting with a plate and glass divided into five food groups.[27]

- 30 percent grains,
- 30 percent vegetables
- 20 percent fruits
- 20 percent protein
- accompanied by a smaller circle representing dairy, such as a glass of low-fat/nonfat milk or a yogurt cup.

The problem with these suggestions, and most suggestions, is that they don't take into account biological individuality. Taking one of the USDA's recommendations as an example: There are some people who, if they consumed the amount of grains suggested (30% of each meal), would contend with blood sugar dysregulation and insulin resistance and the unending, cascading effects of these serious health challenges. And as it turns out, insulin resistance is the largest problem resulting from the Standard American Diet.

I prefer the Bauman's Eating For Health Plan because it is not a one-size-fits-all diet. The Eating For Health framework emphasizes a wide variety of whole, high-quality foods. High-quality means organic, unrefined, seasonal, and local — whenever possible. The ratio of macronutrients — carbohydrates, proteins, and fats — will depend on an individual's health goals, nutritional status, stressors, life stage, and even the time of year. What's important is the variety; this ensures adequate intake of all vitamins, minerals, and phytonutrients available abundantly in whole foods and necessary for all metabolic processes.

For carbohydrates, whole foods come in the form of crunchy or non-starchy vegetables, leafy vegetables, starchy vegetables, grains, and fruit. Proteins can come from both plants and animals. Animal foods should not only be organic but also from animals raised on species-appropriate diets. For plant proteins, proper preparation (e.g., soaking beans, sprouting grains) is a way to aid in their digestion and obtain the most nutrition out of them. Fats from whole foods such as nuts and seeds, avocados, olives, and coconut are best; high-quality unrefined oils are also fine in small amounts. "Booster foods" such as spices, nutritional yeast, lacto-fermented foods, seaweed and algae are also highlighted in this framework because they are energizing and nutrient dense, and often needed after transitioning away from a Standard American Diet. Finally, hydration plays a vital role in our health and is best achieved via clean water, homemade broths, fresh diluted juices, and a variety of teas.[28]

EATING FOR HEALTH

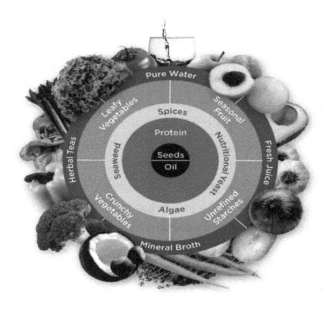

EATING FOR HEALTH SERVING CHART

Food Group	Seeds/Oils	Protein	Leafy Vegetables	Crunchy Vegetables	Unrefined Starches	Seasonal Fruit	Booster Foods
Daily Servings	2-3	2-4	2-3	2-3	2-4	2-4	2-4
Serving Size	1 Tbs oil 2 Tbs seeds	3 oz animal 6 oz vegetable	1 cup	½ cup	½ cup whole grain, 1 medium root vegetable	½ cup or 1 medium piece	1 tsp to 1 Tbs
Examples	flax, sunflower, sesame, almonds	poultry, fish, eggs, milk, beans	salad mix, spinach, kale	broccoli, string beans, onions, celery	grains, bread, yams, winter squash, corn, millet, rice	berries, apple, grape, citrus	nutritional yeast, algae, spices, seaweed

© 2016 Bauman College | Created by Dr. Ed Bauman

Source: https://baumancollege.org/eating-for-health/[29]

Insulin Resistance and Diet

The largest problem with the standard American diet nowadays is that it causes insulin resistance. Insulin resistance is the precursor to pre-diabetes, and diabetes.

Insulin resistance arises from eating too much sugar and carbs.

The steps from high sugar/carb diet to diabetes are these:

- We eat too much sugar and carbs.
- There is excess sugar in the blood. The excess sugar in the bloodstream is toxic. The body needs to get it out of the blood.
- Insulin rises to get the sugar out of the blood. Sugar is stored in the cells under the influence of Insulin.
- Sugar is toxic to the cells, so the cells send signals to the cell membrane to not allow sugar to come in. This is the basis for insulin resistance.
- To overcome this resistance, the body secretes even more insulin to force more sugar into the cells.

This vicious cycle continues until the cells cannot take in anymore sugar at all.

Once the cells cannot take in anymore sugar, blood sugar spikes and we have pre-diabetes. and diabetes.

What happens to this excess sugar inside the cells? Some of it is turned into metabolically active fat and damages any organs it is stored in. Then, the sugar creates oxidative stress. Oxidation is the process by which metals rust. So our cells are oxidizing, rusting in a sense, and eventually becoming extremely dysfunctional.

If you use insulin or diabetes medications, it makes the problem worse. These medications push more sugar into the cells, making blood sugar numbers better but actually, the diabetic metabolic complications are worse.

Dr. Jason Fung's Book, The Diabetes Code uses the analogy of hiding garbage under your bed. Your house looks clean, but it is not. You hide it everywhere out of sight but eventually it will start to rot and smell…until you throw it out.[30]

What he means by throw it out, is that we have to get the excess glucose out of the body. Medications do not do that. That is why Diet and Lifestyle are so important.

We can prove that Type 2 Diabetes is reversible. It is not the chronic, progressive disease as Conventional Medicine portrays it.

We have all experienced people, friends and loved ones who go on low carb diets, lose 25, 30, 50 pounds and their diabetes resolves. All their markers return to normal. As their metabolic markers normalize, they are able to reduce and get off their medication. All their markers return to normal, showing it is possible to reverse Type 2 Diabetes.

Holistic Approach to Diet

So what should you eat? It depends on many factors, such as your health history, your current symptoms or health challenges, your potential nutrient deficiencies (as determined by your doctor or nutrition consultant), your genetic risk factors, medications and other information. Nutrition for you won't look like optimal nutrition for everyone, and this is why most people are so confused about what to eat. Hardly a day goes by without some headline touting the risks or benefits of a particular food. Each of these articles is probably valid for a small percentage of the population and should be ignored by the rest! To understand your own individual dietary needs, a holistic professional will take into account the variables mentioned above as well as address your digestion and gut health, potential food sensitivities, potential hormone imbalances, possible blood sugar dysregulation, the status of your immune and detoxification systems, your long-term health goals, and much more.

Effective Diet Plans

To add to the collective confusion, numerous diet plans are put out into the world on a regular basis. The ones I believe to be effective and worth mentioning share these:

- They contain limited sugars and carbs, and only in the form of a variety of whole, real foods
- They include adequate protein from clean sources
- They contain a variety of healthful fats
- They allow individuals to tailor them to their specific need to prevent inflammation, which is the underlying mechanism of most chronic illness
- Fiber

A word or two about Fiber

Fiber is a type of indigestible carbohydrate found mainly in fruits, vegetables, whole grains, and legumes. In addition to keeping you regular, it offers many other health benefits as well, especially for people with diabetes or pre-diabetes.[31]

A number of studies have found that a high intake of total fiber, from foods and supplements, lowers the risk of heart disease.[32] According to the CDC, the health benefits of fiber include:[33]

- Control your blood sugar. Because the body is unable to absorb and break down fiber, it doesn't cause a spike in blood sugar the way other carbohydrates can. This can help keep your blood sugar in your target range.
- Protect your heart. Fiber prevents your body from taking in some fat and cholesterol, lowering your triglyceride and cholesterol levels (soluble fiber binds to and ushers excess cholesterol out of the body) to help reduce your risk of heart disease.
- Maintain your digestive health. Fiber acts like a scrub brush, cleaning your digestive tract. It helps clean out bacteria and other buildup to improve gut health and help reduce your risk of colon cancer.
- Keep you feeling full and help with weight management.

We need 22-34 grams of fiber a day and can get it naturally by eating whole grains, beans/legumes, non-starchy vegetables, fruits, nuts, and seeds.

Fiber supplements should only be necessary if you can't get your daily requirement via your meals.

If you do decide to increase your fiber intake (via food or supplements) do it slowly. If you increase it too fast, it can cause bloating, gas, constipation, diarrhea, or cramps. Additionally, drink plenty of water to assist moving everything through your system.

To help you find the right diet plan for you, I want to talk about some plans in particular that I have found to be especially beneficial to the heart and brain (and not just the waistline).

The Mediterranean Diet[34]

Many people have studied the Mediterranean Diet. Studies note the low incidence of cardiovascular disease in traditional Mediterranean communities (especially Greece and Southern Italy).

The basis of the Mediterranean Diet are:

- Olive oil (as the main source of added fat)
- Plant foods (cereals, fruits, vegetables, legumes, tree nuts, and seeds)
- Moderate consumption of fish, seafood, and dairy
- Low-to-moderate alcohol (mostly red wine) intake
- Limited use of red meat and other meat products

Not only has it been shown to have positive effects on cardiovascular health, it has also been shown to have positive effects on:

- Metabolic syndrome
- Obesity

- Type 2 diabetes mellitus
- Cancer
- Neurodegenerative diseases

Despite all its proven positive benefits, it has been hard to export this diet to the rest of the world much less keep it alive in Mediterranean countries due to the erosion of traditions and cultures.

Ketogenic Diet (aka, Keto)[35]

Keto is a very-low-carbohydrate and high-fat diet that has proven to be very effective for rapid weight loss. A ketogenic diet primarily consists of high fats, moderate proteins, and very low carbohydrates. These are broken up as shown below:

- 55%-60% fat
- 30%-35% protein
- 5%-10% carbohydrates

In contrast, the average American Diet consists of approximately 55% carbohydrates.

Russel Wilder first used the ketogenic diet to treat pediatric epilepsy in 1921. It only fell out of favor with the introduction of anti-epileptic agents. More recently, the ketogenic diet has reemerged as a means for rapid weight loss.

The key to Keto is the extreme limitation of carbohydrates (less than 50g per day). They are the primary source of energy production for the body. Without carbohydrates, insulin secretion is reduced and glucose is used up. To compensate, ketone bodies (a super fuel) are produced to provide energy to the heart, muscle tissue, and kidneys.

Overweight individuals with metabolic syndrome, insulin resistance, and type 2 diabetes are likely to see improvements in the clinical markers of disease risk. Glucose control improves due to less glucose introduction and improved insulin sensitivity. In addition to reducing weight, especially truncal obesity and insulin resistance, low-carb diets also may help improve:

- Blood pressure
- Blood glucose regulation
- Triglycerides
- HDL cholesterol levels
- LDL cholesterol may increase on this diet.

Also, in various studies, the ketogenic diet has shown promising results in a variety of neurological disorders, like:

- Epilepsy
- Dementia
- ALS
- Traumatic brain injury (TBI)

And can also help in:

- Acne
- Cancer
- Metabolic disorders

You cannot stay on a ketogenic diet for more than 6-12 months, primarily because you won't be able to consume an adequate amount of much-needed phytonutrients from colorful vegetables and fruits. Additionally, to be effective, it must be done for a minimum of 2 to 3 weeks. You must closely monitor your renal functions while on the diet. Finally, the transition from a ketogenic diet to a standard diet should be gradual and well-controlled.

Paleo Diet[36]

The paleo diet is modeled on prehistoric human diets. It typically includes foods that could be obtained by hunting or gathering such as lean meats, fish, fruits, vegetables, nuts, and seeds. The paleo diet excludes foods common to farming – which humans didn't eat prior to the Agricultural Revolution roughly 12,000 years ago – such as dairy, legumes, and grains. The idea behind the diet is that we are genetically mismatched to modern food (most especially when it is processed), which contributes to obesity, diabetes, and heart disease.

In general, paleo diets follow these guidelines.

What to eat

- Fruits
- Vegetables
- Nuts and seeds
- Lean meats, especially grass-fed animals or wild game
- Fish, especially those rich in omega-3 fatty acids, such as salmon, mackerel and albacore tuna
- Oils from fruits and nuts (e.g., olive oil or walnut oil)

What to avoid

- Grains (e.g., wheat, oats and barley)
- Legumes (e.g., beans, lentils, peanuts and peas)
- Dairy
- Refined sugar
- Salt
- Potatoes
- Highly processed foods

The diet also emphasizes hydration and physical activity.

Proponents of the Paleo diet claim it leads to:

- Weight loss
- Improved glucose tolerance
- Blood pressure control
- Lower triglycerides
- Appetite management

There are concerns about the Paleo diet as it excludes good sources of fiber, vitamins and nutrients (from grains and legumes) and protein and calcium (from dairy).

Daniel Fast Diet[37]

The Daniel Fast diet is a 10-21 day dietary modification plan emphasizing simplicity and plant-based nutrition inspired by the character of Daniel in the Bible. In the Bible, Daniel is directed to a strict diet for 10 days with positive physical, intellectual, and spiritual outcomes. Many people now use it as a temporary, short-term fast or "detox" from modern food and lifestyle.[38]

The Daniel Fast diet consists of non-energy-restricted choices of foods from plant sources, minimally processed and prepared in a healthy and simple way.

Foods to eat[39]

Here are foods that are approved while on the Daniel Fast:

- **Beans and lentils.** All types are permitted.
- **Nuts and seeds.** All types are permitted, except those with added salt.
- **Fruits and vegetables.** All types are permitted.
- **Oils and fats.** Only vegetable oils are allowed, and only in small amounts, such as to sauté vegetables.
- **Whole grains.**
- **Unleavened bread.** Whole grain breads and flat-breads made without yeast, sugars, or preservatives are permitted.
- **Herbs and spices.** All fresh and dried herbs and spices are permitted and encouraged as flavor enhancers, though salt should be used sparingly.
- **Beverages.** Water should be your main beverage. Unsweetened plant beverages such as 100% fruit juice are permitted in small amounts.
- **Vitamins and supplements.** All are permitted as needed.

Foods to avoid

Here are foods that should be avoided on the diet:

- **Meat, poultry, fish, and eggs.**
- **Dairy products.** All dairy should be avoided.
- **Added sugar and artificial sweeteners.**
- **Yeast.** Yeast and leavened bread products are not permitted.
- **Refined grains.** White flour and white rice are not permitted.
- **Processed foods.** Any food that is heavily processed or contains added colors, flavors, or preservatives should be avoided.
- **Solid fats.** Butter, ghee, lard, margarine, and shortening should be avoided.
- **Certain beverages.** Alcohol, coffee, tea, kombucha, soda, and sugar-sweetened beverages should be avoided.

The Daniel Fast is not considered a weight loss diet. In studies, it has been shown to improves several risk factors for metabolic and cardiovascular disease such as reductions in total and LDL cholesterol, systolic and diastolic blood pressure, and trends for reductions in insulin, HOMA-IR, and C-reactive protein.[40]

Vegetarian and Vegan Diets[41]

The final diet plan(s) I want to talk about are also plant-based diets. A vegetarian diet excludes meat. A vegan diet further excludes animal products (e.g., milk and eggs)

Plant-only diets carry some risk of inadequate protein, vitamin, and mineral intake. These diets come with the increased risk of not obtaining good fats or protein without also getting unnecessary/unwanted carbohydrates. This, in turn, may create a substantive pitfall for those individuals who need animal foods to maintain blood sugar regulation, which is at the core of a healthy metabolism. But for others, these risks are readily overcome by choosing the right vegetarian foods and, when necessary, supplements.

Research shows that eating more fruits, vegetables, grains, and beans, and avoiding meat, dairy products, and eggs—which are packed with saturated fat and cholesterol—is the best prescription for blood pressure control and cholesterol management. Studies have found that a plant-based diet:[42]

- Reduces the risk of death from cardiovascular disease by 40 percent.
- Reduces the risk of coronary heart disease by 40 percent.
- Fully or partially opens blocked arteries in up to 91 percent of patients.
- Reduces the risk of hypertension, by 34 percent.
- Is associated with 29 mg/dL and 23 mg/dL lower total cholesterol and LDL-C levels, respectively, compared with non-vegetarian diets.

Vegan Diet

The Vegan Diet is another Diet that has become more popular. Some people choose this diet because they believe it is moral to avoid animal products, and they also believe it is healthier and better for the environment.[43]

While not questioning people's moral or environmental choices, I would like to speak to the health issue.

If anyone has Insulin Resistance, Pre-diabetes or Diabetes, a Vegan Diet is difficult. Most of the plant protein comes with carbohydrate, so it makes it difficult to improve Insulin Resistance and reverse the diabetes and pre-diabetes.

There have been studies that show people's health improving when they compare people following a Vegan Diet to the general population. Studies showed decreased mortality amongst the vegans.[44] However, people who choose a Vegan Diet are often more health conscious. These studies had not controlled for other Lifestyle behaviors such as smoking and exercise. And they were comparing them to the general population with no control on the type of diet that is typically high carb and full of unhealthy fat. That's comparing apples to oranges.

But what happens if they compare them to meat eaters who are health conscious? Who exercise and eat a lower carb diet? The term "Nutrivore" was coined for these health-conscious omnivores. These studies paint a different picture. The mortality difference seen when comparing Vegans to the general population disappeared when comparing Vegans to Nutrivores.[45]

Bottom line, while someone may choose to be a Vegan for many reasons, health should not be the primary driver since you can live as long as a healthy Nutrivore as a Vegan. And, taking health struggles and biologic individuality into account, being a Nutrivore could be a healthier diet choice for some.

Attention Deficit / Hyperactivity Disorder (AD/HD) Diet[46]

The key to an AD/HD Diet is to get the right foods and avoid the wrong one. The goal is to improves focus, decrease hyperactivity and generally avoid spikes and lulls in blood sugar.

The average meal for someone with AD/HD should be:

- 50% Fruits and Vegetables
- 25% Lean Protein (e.g., lean beef, pork, poultry, fish, eggs, beans, nuts, soy, and low-fat dairy products)
- 25% Carbohydrates (e.g., whole grains)

Foods to be avoided if you have AD/HD include:

- High sugar foods and snacks
- Artificial Dyes and Preservatives
- Foods that cause allergies (e.g., gluten, wheat, corn, and soy)

Vitamins and Minerals for you AD/HD Diet

- Zinc, Iron, and Magnesium
- B Vitamins (e.g., B-6)
- Multivitamins
- Omega-3 Fatty Acids (e.g., sardines, tuna, and salmon)
- Ginkgo and Ginseng

The Autoimmune Protocol (AIP) Diet[47]

People with autoimmune disease have faulty immune systems. Instead of creating antibodies to fight foreign or bad cells, they create antibodies that attack healthy cells. This leads to disorders like lupus, inflammatory bowel disease (IBD) , celiac disease, type 1 diabetes, psoriasis, and rheumatoid arthritis.

The Autoimmune Protocol (AIP) aims to reduce inflammation, pain, and other symptoms caused by autoimmune diseases.

Some research has shown that certain foods (e.g., gluten) can increase intestinal permeability (aka, Leaky Gut) which can lead to autoimmune disease. However, sometimes it works the other way around, whereby intestinal permeability prompts food sensitivities. Either way, a prerequisite for all AI conditions is intestinal permeability. Accordingly, a goal of AIP is to eliminate foods that may be causing gut inflammation, leaky gut, and systemic inflammation, and replace them with nutritious foods that heal the gut, thereby reducing the symptoms (i.e., inflammation and pain) of autoimmune disease.

The AIP diet is much like the Paleo diet, but stricter. It is conducted in two phases. First you eliminate everything that might be causing you issues, including:

- Grains,
- Legumes
- Nuts
- Seeds
- Nightshade vegetables
- Eggs

- Dairy
- Tobacco
- Alcohol
- Coffee
- Oils
- Food additives
- Refined and processed sugars
- Certain medications (e.g., non-steroidal anti-inflammatory drugs (NSAIDs)

Once your body has stabilized, foods can be added back one at a time to determine which ones your body can handle and which ones are causing you issues.

AIP has been shown to be an effective part of a Multi-disciplinary, Supported Lifestyle Intervention for Hashimoto's Thyroiditis based on the improved Quality of Life as measured by the patient's Medical Symptom Questionnaire, and for some, lowered the amount of thyroid medication they need.[48]

Foods that support Women's Hormone Balance

Foods that support hormone balance for women include those that support detoxification, adrenal health, thyroid function, and gut health. Colorful, antioxidant-rich plant foods as well as its adaptogens, fiber and healthy fats are important for women's reproductive health.

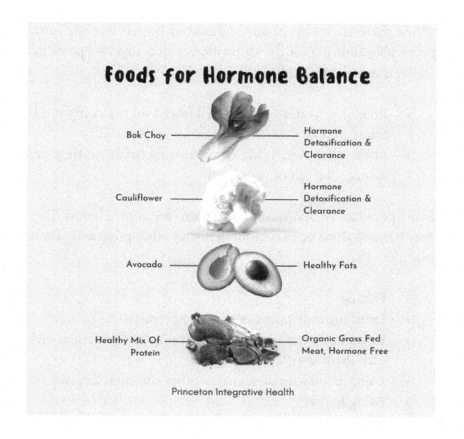

Foods for Hormone Balance

Bok Choy — Hormone Detoxification & Clearance

Cauliflower — Hormone Detoxification & Clearance

Avocado — Healthy Fats

Healthy Mix Of Protein — Organic Grass Fed Meat, Hormone Free

Princeton Integrative Health

Detox[49]

A detox is your opportunity to give your body a break and allow you own self-cleaning and self-healing processes to kick into gear
~mesha_healthylife

In addition to the Daniel Plan, there are a variety of "detoxification" diets, regimens, and therapies—sometimes called "detoxes" or "cleanses". Proponents have suggested them as ways to remove toxins from your body, lose weight, and/or promote health.

When there are toxins in our bodies, our bowels become more permeable allowing for the absorption of non-digested proteins. Detox is done in two phases:[50]

- Phase 1 activates toxins by making fat soluble compounds water soluble
- Phase 2 involves safely encapsulating toxins so they can be excreted out of your body

Some popular "Detoxification" programs are shown below. They may be used alone or in conjunction with other programs. These include:

- Fasting
- Drinking only juices or similar beverages
- Eating only certain foods, oftentimes phytonutrient-rich carbohydrates
- Using dietary supplements or other commercial products
- Using herbs
- Cleansing the colon (lower intestinal tract) with enemas, laxatives, or colon hydrotherapy (also called "colonic irrigation" or "colonics")
- Reducing environmental exposures
- Using a sauna.

During Detoxes, you may lose weight due to reduced caloric intake. The key is to keep monitoring your intake after completion of the cleanse so you don't just readd the calories.

Intermittent Fasting[51]

Where most diets are concerned with what you eat, fasting is focused on when you eat. When fasting, you switch between eating and not eating on a schedule. In this way, your body burns what you have eaten and then pulls from your fat stores. The goal of fasting is to help manage your weight (as fasting could prevent over consuming calories) and prevent, or even reverse, some diseases.

There tends to be a 2–4-week adjustment period when you start fasting. During that time, you may feel hungry and cranky (i.e., "hangry"). After that time, your body should get used to the new regime and normalize.

Another thing to watch is what you eat when you do eat. The goal is to eat normally. Mainly, don't eat too much or food with little to no nutritional value.

Many things happen during intermittent fasting that can protect organs against chronic diseases like type 2 diabetes, heart disease, age-related neurodegenerative disorders, even inflammatory bowel disease and many cancers. Some of the benefits of fasting that research has found so far:

- Thinking and memory.
- Heart health (blood pressure and resting heart rates as well as other heart-related measurements)
- Physical performance
- Diabetes and obesity
- Tissue health

Like all major changes, be sure to talk to your doctor before starting to fast.

Organic[52]

Regardless of which diet plan you use, consider using only organic and organically raised ingredients. The U.S. Department of Agriculture sets specification for a product or animal to be grown or raised to in order to be considered "organic". For agricultural products, these requirements include non-use of hormones, pesticides, irradiation or bio-engineering. Animals used for meat, poultry, eggs or dairy products must not receive antibiotics or growth hormones. Additionally, organic products are subject to the same USDA safety standards as all other food products.

Organic advocates argue that organic products are more nutritious, taste better, and safer to eat. Regardless, products are usually fresher due to the lack of preservatives.

Here's my simple rule: Eat more organic, proper macronutrients, more veggies and fruit. For more guidance, the Environmental Working Group publishes a list called "The Dirty Dozen" each year[53]:

https://www.ewg.org/foodnews/dirty-dozen.php

Genetically Modified Organisms (GMO)

Currently, over 90% of corn and soy in the United States is GMO. There are not many long-term studies of the possible negative effects related to human consumption of GMOs but the Institute for Responsible Technology and The Environmental Working Group, "have found an alarming number of connections between GMOs and health problems, including intestinal damage, inflammation, higher rates of disease, and even death" "particularly if you have an autoimmune or inflammatory condition".[54] Additionally, they may cause allergic reactions (to themselves or other foods) and they may increase antibiotic resistance.[55]

- GMOs Contain More Pesticides than Non-GMOs
- GMOs were developed to allow for more herbicides
- Genetically Modified Foods Cause Leaky Gut
- GMOs create their own insecticides that also have negative effects on the human digestive system, namely, leaky gut, which is a precursor to autoimmune disease
- GMOs Disrupt Your Gut Balance
- The additional pesticides used adversely affect good gut bacteria while not affecting bad gut bacteria thereby causing an imbalance

Despite the potential positives, I feel the negative effects are far more damaging to us. Therefore, I recommend avoiding them. The easiest way to ensure that you are not getting GMO food is to only eat 100% organic. Additionally, only grass-fed meat to ensure it has not been fed GMO corn or soy.[56]

Diet and Supplements

Before we actually discuss supplements, I want to touch briefly on Macronutrients and overall dietary plans.

When people discuss Diets and Dietary plans, they are discussing varying the ratio and quantity of macronutrients. Macronutrients are fat, protein and carbohydrates. For example, the Ketogenic Diet is a dietary plan that is much higher in fats than carbohydrates in order to create the ketotic state. The Standard American Diet has a much higher percentage of calories from carbohydrates and sugar than the Ketogenic Diet.

But it is not just the ratio of the macronutrients that makes different diets…well, different. It is the actual foods we put into them. It is the proportion of whole foods to processed foods.

I want to reemphasize here the importance of eating a primarily whole food-based diet. We should be able to get the majority, if not always all, of our nutrients from a rich, varied and delicious whole foods diet. Processing foods removes many of these nutrients. The more processed food we eat, the less nutrient rich our diets will be.

Nutrient Classes

The major classes of nutrients are the macronutrients and the micronutrients. The macronutrients, the fat, carbohydrate and protein (which is built from amino acids) make up the bulk of the nutrients and calories of our diets.

The micronutrients, the fat-soluble and water-soluble vitamins, the major and minor minerals are also critical to our health.

The seven major minerals include calcium, phosphorus, magnesium, sodium, potassium, chloride and sulfur.

The nine trace minerals are chromium, copper, fluoride, iodine, iron, manganese, molybdenum, selenium and zinc.

The water-soluble vitamins are Vitamin C and the B Vitamins.

The fat-soluble vitamins are Vitamins A,D,E and K.

Sometimes people do not get all the nutrients they need from food, especially the micronutrients. That could be related to internal factors such as inflammation or malabsorption. Or it could be related to external factors such as mineral depleted soil.

Supplements are supplemental, but sometimes needed.

As I mentioned above, we should get the majority of our nutrients from a whole foods, versus processed foods, diet. However, sometimes you may have some nutritional gaps that need to be filled. Many people will do this with a high-quality multivitamin.

Sometimes people have health challenges and need higher doses of a particular vitamin or mineral. People with osteoporosis often need supplemental Vitamin D and calcium for example.

While the benefits of using these various supplements and therapies is beyond the scope of this book, the best thing you can do is find a Practitioner conversant in Nutritional Therapy and work with them. We are often measuring levels of specific vitamins or doing a Micronutrient test. I will discuss the most common supplements I recommend to people below.

Vitamin D:

Vitamin D, while called a vitamin, is actually a pro-hormone. It is activated by two protein enzyme hydroxylation steps, the first in the liver and the second in the kidneys. Because people do not get enough sunlight to generate Vitamin D Production in the skin, people are often deficient. The standard levels of Vitamin D are 30-100, but there is evidence that levels above 50 are more beneficial.[57]

While Vitamin D is mostly known for its bone health properties, preventing rickets and preventing and treating osteoporosis, it has myriad of other functions. Vitamin D is critical to healthy bones since your body can only absorb calcium when it is present. Vitamin D also has anti-inflammatory, antioxidant and neuroprotective properties that support immune health, muscle function and brain cell activity.[58] Low vitamin D levels are associated with increased overall and cardiovascular mortality, cancer incidence and mortality, and autoimmune diseases such as multiple sclerosis.[59]

From the Harvard School of Public Health:[60]

> "Laboratory studies show that vitamin D can reduce cancer cell growth, help control infections and reduce inflammation. Many of the body's organs and tissues have receptors for vitamin D, which suggest important roles beyond bone health, and scientists are actively investigating other possible functions."

In this article, they present research that supports its use for:

- Bone Health and muscle strength
- Cancer
- Heart disease (Which, after all, is the most important muscle in the body)
- Diabetes
- Immune function and autoimmune conditions
- Reducing overall mortality

The recommended daily amount (RDA) of vitamin D is 600 international units (IU) for people ages 1 to 70. The RDA is meant to prevent rickets. More Vitamin D is needed, especially if you are not getting the sunshine you need. Vitamin D isn't naturally found in many foods, but you can get it from:

- Fortified milk
- Fortified cereal
- Fatty fish (e.g., salmon, mackerel and sardines)
- Your body also makes Vitamin D when exposed to direct sunlight (UV); it converts a chemical in your skin into an active form of the vitamin (calciferol)

Vitamin D and COVID-19:

My feeling about Vitamin D and COVID-19 is this: Some studies indicate that Vitamin D levels before contracting COVID can be a factor in the severity of disease. People with the lowest levels appear to be more at risk of severe illness.[61] People with Vit D levels below 50 are more likely to require hospitalization, critical care and have higher mortality than those with Vitamin D levels above 50.

COVID can cause critical illness. Vitamin D can potentially be helpful. Downsides are very small, especially when levels are being checked. I previously stated in the COVID section of Chapter 3 that I recommend Vitamin D supplementation to my patients, anywhere from 1,000 IU to 5,000 IU, to achieve a level between 50 – 80 ng/ml, higher than many conventional recommendations. If people get enough sunlight, they may not need supplementation, but I find this is rare. I do not feel it is the only factor to prevent severe COVID, but it is an easily controllable factor.[62][63]

Vitamin C

Although Vitamin C (also known as ascorbic acid) is not produced by the human body it is critical to growth, development and repair of body tissues.[64] It does this because, an antioxidant, it protect your body against free radicals. Vitamin C also helps your body absorb and store iron. The benefits of Vitamin C include:[65]

- Wound healing
- Cardiovascular health
- Cataracts and age-related macular degeneration
- Diabetes
- Anemia
- Pollution
- Allergies
- Motion sickness

The official daily recommendation for Vitamin C is 75mg for women and 90mg for men.[66] I personally recommend people take 1,000 to 2,000 mg a day. People will know if they are taking too much because it will cause diarrhea. Since it only comes your diet, you must ensure you eat the right foods.[67]

- Citrus fruits
- Berries
- Potatoes
- Tomatoes
- Red and green peppers
- Cabbage
- Brussels sprouts
- Broccoli
- Spinach

If you are unable to get enough via diet alone, you can get Vitamin C via supplements.

Calcium

Calcium is a mineral most often associated with healthy bones and teeth, although it also plays an important role in blood clotting, helping muscles to contract, and regulating normal heart rhythms and nerve functions.[68]

We need about 1000-1200 mg of calcium a day for healthy living. The benefits of getting enough Calcium are: [69]

- Lower Blood Pressure
- Increased Bone Health
- Decreased Risk of Colorectal Cancer
- Decreased Risk of Kidney Stones

Calcium supplements are not an adequate replacement of milk and other dairy products since milk naturally provides nutrients such as protein, vitamin B2 and B12 and minerals including calcium, phosphorus, potassium and iodine.[70] Calcium can also be found in Winter Squash, Edamame, Almonds, and leafy greens.

If you take Calcium for Bone Health, it is often best to take make sure you have adequate Magnesium in your diet.

Magnesium[71]

Without Magnesium, Vitamin D and Calcium supplements may be ineffective. You need the Magnesium to help with metabolic activities.

Magnesium is important for:

- Heart and Blood Vessel Health
- GI Health
- Brain Health
- Bone Health

However, studies estimate that most of the population does not get adequate Magnesium intake. The recommended allowance for magnesium for males is 420 mg per day and 320 mg per day for females. However, the standard diet in the United States contains only approximately 50% of that, meaning a large portion of the population is Magnesium deficient.

Turmeric

Turmeric comes from a tall plant that grows in Asia and Central America. It is a major ingredient in Curry. The active ingredient in Turmeric, Curcumin, has powerful biological properties. Turmeric and Curcumin are amongst Nature's most powerful anti-inflammatory compounds. It has been used in Indian medicine for over 3000 years.[72] The positive side effects of Turmeric are below:[73]

- It's anti-inflammatory
- It can relieve pain
- It improves liver function
- It may help reduce the risk of cancer
- It can aid your digestion

Recommended doses are 500-2000mg per day. The most common way to take Turmeric is via an extract, but you can also certainly use it in cooking if it fits your palate.

Essential Fatty Acids: Omega 3s[74]

The three main omega-3 fatty acids are alpha-linolenic acid (ALA), eicosapentaenoic acid (EPA), and docosahexaenoic acid (DHA). ALA is found mainly in plant oils such as flaxseed, soybean, and canola oils. DHA and EPA are found in fish and other seafood. Your body can convert a small amount of ALA into DHA and EPA but the primary source for all three is what you eat and drink.

Omega-3s help make up the membranes that surround each cell in your body and affect the function of the cell receptors in these membranes. They provide the basis for making hormones that regulate blood clotting, contraction and relaxation of artery walls, and inflammation.[75] DHA levels are especially high in the retina (eye), brain, and sperm cells. Omega-3s also provide calories to give your body energy and have many functions in your heart, blood vessels, lungs, immune system, and endocrine system (the network of hormone-producing glands).

I recommend supplements of Omega-3 Fatty Acids because they are anti-inflammatory and can lower elevated triglycerides. Benefits include:[76]

- Reduced risk of cardiovascular disease.
- Reduced risk of death if you have cardiovascular disease.
- Reduced risk of sudden cardiac death caused by an abnormal heart rhythm
- Reduced risk of blood clots because omega-3 fatty acids help prevent blood platelets from clumping together
- Keeping the lining of the arteries smooth and free of damage that can lead to thick, hard arteries. This helps keep plaque from forming in the arteries
- Lowering triglyceride levels by slowing the rate they form in the liver. High levels of triglycerides in the blood increase the risk of heart disease
- Less inflammation. Atherosclerosis (hardening of the arteries) is thought to involve your body's inflammatory response. Omega-3 fatty acids slow production of substances that are released during the inflammatory response
- Raise levels of high-density lipoprotein (HDL/"good" cholesterol)
- Lower blood pressure. People who eat fish tend to have lower blood pressure than those who don't

There is no recommended daily allowance for DHA or EPA. For ALA, the recommended daily allowance is 1.6g for men and 1.1g for women.

The best sources of Omega-3s are the following foods:

- Fish and other seafood (i.e., salmon (wild caught), mackerel, tuna, herring, anchovies and sardines)
- Tuna, swordfish and shark are high in Omega-3s, but also high in Mercury. These fish should be consumed sparingly.
- Nuts and seeds (e.g., flaxseed, chia seeds, and walnuts)
- Plant oils (e.g., flaxseed, soybean, and canola oil)
- Fortified foods (e.g., eggs, yogurt, juices, milk, soy beverages, and infant formulas)
- Supplements: Fish oil is the most common way to supplement Omega-3s. Make sure you get high quality fish oil and they are checking for mercury and other heavy metals. For people who are philosophically opposed to fish oil, you can also get Omega-3s from algae oil, krill oil or flaxseed oil.

Eat to live, not live to eat "Salud, chindon"

Remember, in addition to your diet being healthy, to be successful, it must be affordable, available and enjoyable. Otherwise, you will not be able to maintain it, nor may you want to. It is the majority of what you do that will determine your health, not the occasional going off the plan.

I recommend people be flexible, to make choices that bring them joy, especially when celebrating in community with others such as birthdays, weddings and other joyous celebrations. "Salud, chin-don!"— often said at meals, Italian for health for a hundred years.

Drinks

Now that we have talked about food, we need to look at drinks. Studies have shown that adults can go about 3 weeks without food but only about 3 days without water.[77].

Water[78]

Drinking water is like washing out your insides. The water will cleanse the system, fill you up, decrease your caloric load and improve the function of all your tissues.
~Kevin R. Stone

Water is key to maintaining a healthy body and avoiding dehydration. What you probably did not know is the way you drink water plays a role in its absorption in the body.

The question is, "Is there a right or wrong way to drink water?" Surprisingly, there is and you've probably have been doing it wrong.

Optimal Water Drinking:[79]

- About 15.5 cups (3.7 liters) of fluids a day for men
- About 11.5 cups (2.7 liters) of fluids a day for women
- About 20% of daily fluid intake usually comes from food and the rest from drinks
- Sip from a glass—You tend to drink more, remain hydrated and avoid bloating

- Sitting—because when standing or walking, blood flow is primarily towards our arms and legs
- Room Temperature—instead of very cold
- Water should be as pure as possible. Oftentimes, this means filtering the water.
- There are many water filtration systems available

Caffeine

Caffeine is a stimulant that, according the USDA, about 80% of adults consume caffeine every day.[80] Caffeine can aid alertness if used correctly but is not a substitute for alertness and decision making provided by sleep.

Heavy caffeine use on a daily basis may lose its alerting effect. Instead, consider it a "medicine" and use it strategically for its alerting effects.[81]

Too much caffeine can cause severe disturbances to the heart and nervous system.[82] For healthy adults, the FDA has cited 400 milligrams a day—that's about four or five cups of coffee—as an amount not generally associated with dangerous, negative effects.[83] More than that can cause severe disturbances to the heart and nervous system. [84]

Sometimes excess caffeine consumption – especially later in the day – is a proxy for blood sugar imbalance. Oftentimes people turn to a cup of coffee when their energy is running low. Instead, they should investigate what they ate earlier in the day – a culprit for afternoon fatigue is usually refined sugars and carbohydrates. When this is addressed, the need for a cup of coffee typically goes away.

Alcohol

Alcohol is classified as a Central Nervous System Depressant, meaning that it slows down brain functioning and neural activity. Alcohol does this by enhancing the effects of the neurotransmitter GABA. Alcohol can depress the central nervous system so much that it results in impairment such as slurred speech, unsteady movement, disturbed perceptions, and an inability to react quickly. Alcohol reduces an individual's ability to think rationally, lessens inhibitions, and distorts judgment. If an individual consumes too much alcohol too rapidly, they can depress the central nervous system to a point of respiratory failure, coma, or death.[85]

CDC Dietary Guidelines for alcohol[86]

- Alcohol consumption is associated with a variety of short- and long-term health risks, including motor vehicle crashes, violence, sexual risk behaviors, high blood pressure, and various cancers (e.g., breast cancer).
- The risk of these harms increases with the amount of alcohol you drink. For some conditions, like some cancers, the risk increases even at very low levels of alcohol consumption (less than 1 drink).
- To reduce the risk of alcohol-related harms, the *2020-2025 Dietary Guidelines for Americans* recommends that adults of legal drinking age can choose not to drink, or to drink in moderation by limiting intake to 2 drinks or less in a day for men or 1 drink or less in a day for women, on days when alcohol is consumed. The *Guidelines* also do not recommend that individuals who do not drink alcohol start drinking for any reason and that if adults of

legal drinking age choose to drink alcoholic beverages, drinking less is better for health than drinking more.[87]

Sugar-Sweetened Beverages (SSBs)[88]

SSBs include, but are not limited to, regular soda (not sugar-free), fruit drinks, sports drinks, energy drinks, sweetened waters, and coffee and tea beverages with added sugars. SSBs are leading sources of added sugars in the American diet. Frequently drinking sugar-sweetened beverages is associated with weight gain, obesity, type 2 diabetes, heart disease, kidney diseases, non-alcoholic liver disease, tooth decay and cavities, and gout, a type of arthritis. Limiting sugary drink intake can help individuals maintain a healthy weight and have healthy dietary patterns.

There is an even more insidious effect of too much Sugar and Insulin Resistance. Type 2 Diabetes is Insulin Resistance in the cells of the body. But when the Brain develops Insulin Resistance and Cognitive Decline, that has been dubbed Type 3 Diabetes. The Brain is the most energy intense organ in the body. Due to the Insulin Resistance in the Brain cells, they cannot use glucose for an efficient energy source. This results in a poorly functioning brain. That is the reason for a ketogenic type diet—the Brain (and other organs) work much better on ketones when there is significant Insulin Resistance. If you or anyone is at risk for Cognitive Decline, then it is important to take steps to avoid developing Insulin Resistance. It is especially important to avoid Sugar Sweetened Beverages in this context.

Fructose deserves special mention here. Because fructose can only be metabolized in the liver, it is particularly powerful in helping create fatty liver. Soda and some other sweetened beverages contain large amounts of fructose and should be avoided entirely.[89]

When too much fructose reaches the liver, the liver uses the excess to create fat (i.e., lipogenesis). Eventually, people who consume too much fructose can develop non-alcoholic fatty liver disease, a condition in which too much fat is stored in the liver cells.[90] This one of the first steps in Insulin Resistance and the cascade of health problems that follow.

For any other store-bought food, candy, sauce with added sugar, you must read the label to see if it contains fructose. Other foods that could contain fructose are:[91]

- Most fruits, especially dried fruits and fruits canned in juice or syrup. Our bodies are usually able to handle the amount of fructose in fresh fruit.
  - Fruits low in fructose include avocados, bananas, cranberries, cantaloupe, lemons, limes, oranges, pineapple, and strawberries
- Vegetables including artichoke, asparagus, broccoli, leeks, mushrooms, okra, onions, peas, red pepper, shallots and tomato products. Most of the time, we are able to handle the fructose found in fresh vegetables.
- Foods with wheat as the main ingredient
- Sweeteners such as honey, agave nectar and high-fructose corn syrup.
- Sodas and desserts sweetened with fructose.

Diet Soda[92]

Diet drinks with zero sugar and calories were introduced in the 1960s. Now that they are the second most popular drink to coke, you would expect a decrease in obesity and diabetes. That has not happened. In fact, they have found other issues for people consuming diet drinks:

- A 47% increase in obesity
- A 43% increase in vascular events (strokes and heart attacks)

There is even anecdotal evidence that shows eating sweets (even fake ones) makes you crave more sweets. They show little to no benefit and appear to potentially to cause harm if taken in high quantities. Bottom line, artificial sweeteners are not food, they are chemicals. Although they are marketed as a safe alternative to sugar, I don't recommend them.

Sweeteners, not artificial

If you need to use a sweetener, I recommend using natural sweeteners such as small amounts of

- Honey
- Maple Syrup
- Monkfruit
- Stevia

Now that we have talked about food and drink, we have another area to consider, the containers they come in…namely, Plastic.

Plastic[93]

When it comes to food, Plastic is everywhere. It's in our plates, our cutlery, bottles, bags and wraps used to store, cook and serve food and drinks. The question is, how safe is it?

Studies have found that certain chemicals in plastic can leach into the food and beverages we eat/drink. Because some of these chemicals, like BPA, mimic and disrupt our hormones, they have been linked to health problems such as metabolic disorders (including obesity) and reduced fertility. This leaching process can be made worse and occur faster when plastic is exposed to heat. Think about that next time you are microwaving your leftovers. It is recommended that you store and microwave your food in glass containers.

CHAPTER 5

EXERCISE AND ACTIVITY

Lack of activity destroys the good condition of every human being, while movement and methodical physical exercise save it and preserve it.
~Plato

Activity and Exercise

Activity and Exercise has positive benefits to sleep, stress mitigation and Mental Health.

In Chapter two, I stated that you should do 25-30 minutes of moderate activity per day. The good news is you can mix it up between the three main types of exercise:[94]

Aerobic (Cardiovascular Health)[95]

- Running
- Cross Country Skiing
- Swimming
- Running or Jogging
- Outdoor cycling
- Walking

Anerobic (Cardiovascular Health and Strength)[96]

- Weightlifting
- Jumping or Jumping Rope
- Sprinting
- High Intensity Interval Training (HIIT)
- Biking

Stretching (Flexibility and Pain Tolerance)[97]

- Active stretching
- Passive stretching
- Dynamic stretching
- Proprioceptive neuromuscular facilitation (PNF) stretching, which involves table stretching and the help of a certified stretch therapist

The key is to do something. You can vary between the three types based upon how much time you have, what the weather is like or what facilities are available to you that day. Your workouts will also vary with age. Things that we could do in our twenties are not always feasible today.

Cardiac Rehabilitation/Graded Exercises

After a cardiac event, you need to start exercising again. Graded exercises are done walking or running on a treadmill under the supervision of a cardiologist. During testing, they will monitor your heartbeat and blood pressure. There are two types with specific purposes.[98]

Graded Exercise Stress Test

- To diagnose if you have coronary artery disease
- To determine if ischemia (inadequate blood supply) has gotten worse or gone away following treatment
- To detect heart and circulatory problems such as irregular heartbeat, partially blocked arteries or heart attack risk

Graded Exercise Metabolic Stress Test

- To help you set up a safe and effective exercise program
- To measure your respiratory response to exercise
- To assess Pulmonary or Cardiac Disease

Once they determine your heart health, you can start cardiac rehabilitation. These sessions are done in a highly monitored (Vital signs and EKG) environment and involve a brief warm-up and stretching period, followed by 30-40 minutes of aerobic exercise. This can involve treadmill, stationary bicycle, elliptical or rowing machines.[99]

Cardiac rehabilitation helps patients recovering from a cardiac event to return to and maintain an optimal health status while reducing their risk of future cardiovascular events.[100]

The goal is for you to be able to exercise, have sex, dance, run, and play with your Grandkids.

Mind Body Exercises[101]

Mind-body interventions or exercises from the Far East combine body movement, mental focus, and controlled breathing to improve strength, balance, flexibility, and overall health.[102] Mind Body exercises stimulate the parasympathetic nervous system who's main purpose is to conserve energy to be used later and to regulate bodily functions like digestion and urination.[103]

Three of the most popular Mind Body exercises are Tai Chi, Yoga, and Qigong. There are similarities between all three so I recommend you try them and see which one works best for you.

Tai Chi is a combination of Chinese defensive martial art and vital energy circulation, breathing, and stretching techniques. Tai Chi exercise consists of a series of slow/graceful movements with deep and slow diaphragmatic breathings performed while standing. Tai Chi exercise has been shown to have both physical and psychosocial benefits.

Yoga involves a combination of muscular activity (poses) coupled with focus on self-awareness, breathing, and energy. Yoga integrates an individual's physical, mental, and spiritual components to improve physical and mental health, particularly stress related illnesses.

Qigong exercise is practiced to cultivate the balance and harmony of vital energy in the human body. Qigong exercise, like

Tai Chi, consists of breathing techniques with body movement and meditation to attain deep focus and a relaxed state.

CHAPTER 6
SLEEP

Early to bed and early to rise makes a man
healthy, wealthy, and wise
~Benjamin Franklin

A good laugh and a long sleep are the best cures
in the doctor's book.
~Irish Proverb

Sleep[104]

It is recommended that we get 7 to 8 hours of sleep every night. Do we really need that much sleep? In our busy lives, many people push themselves to function with less sleep than that or some people have sleep disorders.

This topic can be a snooze for some people, but let me assure you that once you hear the facts, it will be a real eye-opener!

You would think this area would be easy. All you have to do is unplug and sleep. As we saw in Chapter 2, only 65% of people are getting the recommended amount. Stress, disruptions, work schedules and medical conditions all contribute to lack of sleep. Unfortunately for the other 35%, lack of sleep can lead to attention lapses, reduced cognition, delayed reactions, and mood swings. There are also the secondary effects of drowsiness (e.g., motor vehicle crashes, mistakes at work) which cause injury, disability and death annually.105

Lack of sleep has been linked to a higher risk for certain diseases and medical conditions such as obesity, type 2 diabetes, high blood pressure, heart disease, stroke, poor mental health, depression and early death.

Sleep is critical to you staying healthy. It allows your body and mind to recharge, and your mind, muscles and heart to slow down and recover leaving you refreshed and alert when you wake up. It is crucial to healing as sleep allows the body to grow and repair tissue, bone and muscle.[106] After a good night's sleep, your hormone, energy, and stress levels have all been reset for the new day.[107]

The Autonomic Nervous System

The Autonomic Nervous System has 2 branches: the Sympathetic and the Parasympathetic.

The Sympathetic Nervous System

The Sympathetic Nervous System is involved in the fight or flight response. If our body senses anything it perceives could be dangerous, this response kicks it. Our body is flooded with adrenaline and cortisol. Our heart beats faster, we breathe deeper, glucose is released to our muscles, readying us to fight or flee. This is life-saving when we are or were under direct physical threat such as a saber tooth tiger in days gone by. The Sympathetic Nervous System is meant to deal with acute threats.

In today's world, the Sympathetic Nervous system reacts to a bad boss, a bad relationship, the stress of traffic, political turmoil, COVID etc...whatever you find stressful. If this happens chronically over a long period of time, it can cause elevated Cortisol levels. This impacts our health by making us more prone to sleep disorders, overeating, insulin resistance, anxiety and other health impacts. If it more seriously impacts our mental health, it can also lead to overconsumption of not just food, but of alcohol and drugs. These overconsumptions, as we know, can have disastrous consequences.

If you need help, please seek it out and accept it.

Stress Mitigation and the Parasympathetic Nervous System

We all need to have some way to relieve our tension and stress so we do not feel overwhelmed. This can be as simple as having a hobby, reading a book, exercising. Some people will want or need more structured activities such as a meditation practice, prayer, yoga, tai-chi etc. Others will need formal counseling.

All of these stress mitigation activities impact our Parasympathetic nervous system. As opposed to the Sympathetic nervous system fight or flight reaction, the Parasympathetic nervous system puts the body into a resting and regenerative state. The most Parasympathetic state we have is when we are in deep sleep states. That is when the body best heals, rejuvenates and regenerates.

It is always a balance. We cannot avoid stress. It is a part of everyday life. But we should seek to balance that stress with activities that help us cope, to rejuvenate ourselves, to balance the Sympathetic and the Parasympathetic nervous system. If we do not have stress mitigating activities during the day AND we are not sleeping well, that can put us at higher risk of having Sympathetic nervous system dominance with the risks mentioned above.

Balance is not something you find, it's something you create.
~Jana Kingsford

And that is what we should all be aiming to achieve.

A healthy diet and positive lifestyle habits can help ensure an adequate amount of sleep each night – but for some, chronic lack of sleep may be the first sign of a sleep disorder.

How to fall asleep naturally

The National Sleep Foundation has some simple rules to help you fall asleep naturally.[108]

- Establish a realistic bedtime and stick to it every night, even on the weekends.

- Maintain comfortable temperature settings and low light levels in your bedroom.
- Keep a comfortable sleep environment by ensuring you have the best mattress, best pillows, and best sheets for your sleep preferences and body type.
- Consider a "screen ban" on televisions, computers and tablets, cell phones, and other electronic devices in your bedroom.
- Abstain from caffeine, alcohol, and large meals in the hours leading up to bedtime.
- Refrain from using tobacco at any time of day or night.
- Exercise during the day; this can help you wind down in the evening and prepare for sleep.

Sleep, Pain and Mental Health

Sleep is often disrupted by factors such as chronic pain, depression or anxiety.

Chronic Pain

There is a correlation between chronic pain and sleep. In the general population, 20% of people with chronic pain report insomnia, whereas only 7.4% of people without chronic pain report these sleep issues. In the healthcare system, 90% of the patients for pain management report sleeping issues with 65% identifying as poor sleepers.[109] The most common complaints are overall sleep time and frequently being awakened.[110]

Depression

Depression and sleep issues are closely related. Up to 90% of individuals suffering from depression also report sleep and circadian disruptions.[111] People with insomnia may have a tenfold higher risk of developing depression than people who get a good night's sleep. Among people with depression, 75 percent have trouble falling asleep or staying asleep. The question is, does the depression affect sleep or does the lack of sleep cause depression.[112] Regardless, don't expect treating one will cure the other; Treat both issues simultaneously.

There are many effective treatments for depression including counseling, talk therapy and medications. Cognitive Behavioral Therapy is a problem focused therapy that can treat both the depression and insomnia concurrently.[113]

It is beyond the scope of this book, but if anyone has chronic pain, depression or anxiety causing sleep disruption, then those factors must be dealt with. Seek a licensed professional if you cannot deal with them yourself.

Sleep Supplements

- Melatonin is a natural hormone produced by your brain to help you fall and stay asleep. It is normally produced in response to darkness.114 If you need to sleep when it's not dark out, you can take Melatonin supplements. In addition to improving sleep, melatonin is also involved in managing immune function, blood pressure and cortisol levels, and it acts as an antioxidant.115 Melatonin supplements are okay for a month or two but after that, you should try sleeping without them.116 Refer to the natural ways to help you sleep above.

- Sleeping Pills should only be occasionally or one-time events (shift change, jet lag). Using them every night can lead to dependence and reduced effectiveness.117 Some sleeping pills have been known to cause rebound insomnia, depression, and suicidal thoughts. Other reported effects are sleepwalking, sleep talking, and/or hallucinations.118

Sleep is so important to our health, there is an entire foundation dedicated to improving health and well-being through sleep education and advocacy. **The National Sleep Foundation** (NSF) is committed to advancing excellence in sleep health theory, research and practice[119]. To help with this awareness, they host two annual campaigns a year.

Sleep Awareness Week[120]

Sleep Awareness Week is hosted at the start of Daylight Savings as a call to action for everyone to recognize the importance of sleep as a crucial measure of their overall health.

Sleep Awareness Week is recognized annually as the premier awareness and education campaign for sleep, when the National Sleep Foundation educates and encourages the public to prioritize sleep as a crucial measure of their overall health and well-being

Drowsy Driving Prevention Week[121]

Drowsy Driving Prevention Week (DDPW) is hosted each year the week following the end of Daylight-Saving Time.

The goal is to reduce the number of drivers who drive while sleep deprived. Drowsy driving is responsible for more than 6,400 U.S. deaths annually. Just think of how many live could be save if people would ensure to get the sleep that they need.

As such, NSF encourages everyone to prioritize sleep and drive when alert and refreshed.

Sleep apnea[122]

One of the most common and potentially serious sleep disorders is sleep apnea. It occurs when your breathing starts and stops through your sleep. Two key indicators are loud snoring and waking up tired even after a full night's sleep. You might also find yourself falling asleep driving, at work, or watching TV. You might also be alerted by your partner who can see/hear your apnea while you sleep.

The main types of sleep apnea are:

- Obstructive sleep apnea (the most common) is caused by throat muscles that relax when we sleep.
- Central sleep apnea is caused by improper commands sent from the brain to the muscles that control breathing.
- Complex sleep apnea syndrome (aka treatment-emergent

central sleep apnea) is a combination of the other two types.

Symptoms

The most common signs and symptoms of obstructive and central sleep apneas include:

- Loud snoring
- Episodes in which you stop breathing during sleep
- Gasping for air during sleep
- Awakening with a dry mouth
- Morning headache
- Difficulty staying asleep (insomnia)
- Excessive daytime sleepiness (hypersomnia)
- Difficulty paying attention while awake
- Irritability

Factors that increase the risk of Obstructive sleep apnea include:

- Excess weight
- Larger neck circumference
- A narrowed airway
- Being male
- Being older
- Family history
- Use of alcohol, sedatives or tranquilizers
- Smoking
- Nasal congestion
- Medical conditions. Congestive heart failure, high blood pressure, type 2 diabetes and Parkinson's disease are some of the conditions that may increase the risk of obstructive

sleep apnea. Polycystic ovary syndrome, hormonal disorders, prior stroke and chronic lung diseases, such as asthma, also can increase risk.

Factors that increase the risk of Central sleep apnea

- Being older
- Being male
- Heart disorders
- Using narcotic pain medications
- Stroke

Complications

Sleep apnea is a serious medical condition. Complications can include:

- Daytime fatigue. The fact that you are constantly being awakened makes it almost impossible to get the beneficial effects of sleep. Over time, it exacerbates the normal effects of lack of sleep. This can lead to lack of concentration, falling asleep, and increased accidents. You might also feel moody, angry, or depressed.
- High blood pressure or heart problems. When your blood oxygen drops suddenly it causes increased blood pressure and strain on your cardiovascular system. Obstructive sleep apnea may increase your risk for heart attack, stroke or, irregular heartbeat. Coupled with heart disease, irregular heartbeat could lead to sudden death.
- Type 2 diabetes. Having sleep apnea increases your risk of developing insulin resistance and type 2 diabetes.
- Metabolic syndrome. High blood pressure, abnormal

cholesterol levels, high blood sugar, and increased waist circumference, are all linked to a higher risk of heart disease.

- Complications with medications and surgery. Being sedated for surgery and laying on your back may exacerbate your sleep apnea. You must tell your doctor before surgery so they can monitor your breathing and oxygen levels more closely.
- Liver problems. People with sleep apnea have a higher probability of getting abnormal results on liver function tests, and their livers are more likely to show signs of scarring (non-alcoholic fatty liver disease).

If not for you, get checked for your partner. Your sleep apnea and/or snoring could be stopping them from getting a full night's sleep as well.

CHAPTER 7

STRESS MITIGATION/ MENTAL EMOTIONAL SPIRITUAL HEALTH

A healthy mind breeds a healthy body, and visa versa!
~Zig Ziglar

Mental Emotional Spiritual Health

As I sit down to write today, my heart is heavy. Naomi Judd died yesterday.

From the Judd family, "We lost our beautiful mother to the disease of mental illness."[123]

Why would I include a Chapter about Mental Health in a book about Vibrancy and Vitality?

I include it because it is absolutely Vital. If our Mental and Emotional Health is suffering, we must address this as we must address all the risk factors to our Longevity. Naomi's case illustrates the extreme, but unfortunately not too uncommon tragedy of dying from a Mental Health illness.

I had already been thinking about Mental Health as I was writing. This tragedy drives home the point that we must first and foremost, assess our Mental, and Emotional Health.

Death by unintentional injury, suicide and homicide dominate the leading causes of death from ages 10 – 34.[124] But as Naomi's case Illustrates, mental health deaths can occur across our lifespan.

Mental Health issues are commonly much more insidious. They can manifest in a myriad of ways. We commonly think of drugs, alcohol, addiction. However, it can manifest as eating too much, sabotaging one's health, being a risk taker and causing unintentional injury or even sabotaging one's success.

Mental, emotional, and spiritual struggles can take a toll on our Cardiovascular health, which is the number one cause of death year in and year out.[125]

There are anonymous, online screening tests that can be used if you feel you are struggling with a Mental Health issue. One such tool is from Mental Health America can be found at https://screening.mhanational.org/screening-tools/[126]

Mental Health includes our emotional, psychological, and social well-being. It affects how we think, feel, and act. It also helps determine how we handle stress.[127]

Emotional Health refers to how a person is able to manage their thoughts, feelings, and emotions through the ups and downs of life.[128]

Spiritual Health is your belief or sense of purpose and meaning. It is what gives you a sense of value or worth in your life. It has nothing to do with religious beliefs.[129]

Stress occurs naturally and helps with our fight-or-flight responses. It can improve alertness, performance and boost memory. [130] Problems occur with prolonged stress such as loss of productivity, health problems, and exhaustion.[131] As such, we need to find ways to mitigate it.

According to the CDC, the benefits of lower stress include:[132]

- Better sleep
- Weight Control
- Less muscle tension
- Better mood
- Better relationships

Stress Mitigation

Some suggestions from the CDC to help with stress.[133]

- Take breaks from watching, reading, or listening to news stories, including those on social media
- Take care of yourself. Eat healthy, exercise, get plenty of sleep, and give yourself a break if you feel stressed out
- Take care of your body

- Take deep breaths, stretch, or meditate
- Avoid excessive alcohol, tobacco, and substance use
- Make time to unwind. Try to do some other activities you enjoy.
- Talk to others (parent, friend, counselor, doctor, or pastor) about your concerns. Talk with people you trust about your concerns and how you are feeling. Share your problems and how you are feeling and coping with a parent, friend, counselor, doctor, or pastor.
- Connect with your community- or faith-based organizations.
- Recognize when you need more help.

Hopefully you're starting to see a pattern here. Everything in this book is interrelated. We've talked about a few of these already (diet, exercise, sleep, alcohol). Let's now look at some of the other items on the list.

Meditation[134] —Numerous studies have shown that meditation is an effective stress-management tool, ultimately reprogramming the brain to the extent that meditators end up with more capacity to manage stress when meditation is a consistent, daily practice. In fact, meditation has been scientifically proven to help alleviate stress after just eight weeks of regular practice.

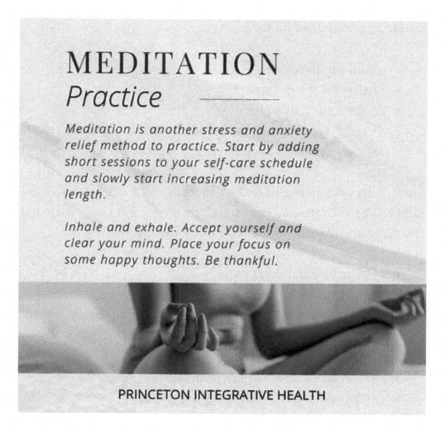

MEDITATION
Practice

Meditation is another stress and anxiety relief method to practice. Start by adding short sessions to your self-care schedule and slowly start increasing meditation length.

Inhale and exhale. Accept yourself and clear your mind. Place your focus on some happy thoughts. Be thankful.

PRINCETON INTEGRATIVE HEALTH

Forest Bathing[135]- Forest bathing and forest therapy (or shin-rin-yoku) developed in Japan in the 1980s. It is a form of mobile meditation where one contemplates every aspect of the forest (sights, sounds, smells). In 1982, Japan made Forest Bathing a part of its national health program. Much research has been done in Japan and South Korea on the diverse health benefits.

Grounding (Earthing)[136] [137][138][139]- Grounding refers to the discovery that bodily contact with the Earth's natural electric charge stabilizes the physiology at the deepest levels. It involves doing activities that "ground" or electrically reconnect you to the earth.

Grounding activities include:

- Walking Barefoot
- Lying on the ground
- Submersing in water
- Using Grounding equipment (mats, sheets/blankets, socks, bands and patches)

Studies are still being done but there is a lot of anecdotal evidence. The overall concept is electrical charges from the earth can have positive effects on your body including:

- Reduces inflammation
- Improves immune response
- Prevention and treatment of chronic inflammatory and autoimmune diseases
- Improves wound healing
- Decreases Chronic pain and stress
- Improves blood flow, energy, and sleep
- Chronic fatigue
- Anxiety and depression
- Sleep disorders
- Cardiovascular disease

Such effects are profound, systemic, and foundational, and often develop rapidly.

Namely, we need to play in the dirt. If not, we lose our tolerance to natural substances. As the world becomes more urbanized and on-line, it is critical that we get back to nature whether it be Grounding or Forest Bathing.

Fun[140]

Go out and have some fun, be silly, enjoy life. Be a child again, forget the responsibilities and pressures of being an adult, regain the wonder and enthusiasm of youth. Why?:

- It gives more energy
- It relieves stress
- It boosts serotonin
- It eliminates depression

Whatever you do, make it social, inclusive, and camaraderie building. Good example of fun activities are sports (watching or playing), games, dancing, karaoke, picnics, dinners, etc.

Heart Rate Variability

Heart rate variability is where the time between your heartbeats fluctuates slightly. This is controlled by your sympathetic:parasympathetic nervous system balance. The higher your sympathetic tone, the less variable your heart rate. The better the balance between your parasympathetic and sympathetic nervous systems, the better your heart rate variability. Many wearable devices such as Fitbit or Oura rings, measure heart rate variability.

There are biofeedback devices that can help people improve heart rate variability. Improving heart rate variability improves sympathetic:parasympathetic balance. This is another powerful tool to help manage stress.

Alright, we talked about what to do about stress, let's now talk about things that we need to add or eliminate from our lifestyles.

CHAPTER 8
LIFESTYLE

A lifestyle change begins with a vision and a single step.
~Jeff Calloway

Nothing we do can be done by itself. Therefore to make any lasting change, we need to look at our overall lifestyle.

The Ornish Program

I put this here because, as it was originally implemented, it encompasses a multiple of "intensive" lifestyle changes. It includes:[141]

- What you eat (less than 10% fat whole-foods vegetarian diet)
- How much you move
- How you manage stress
- How much love and support you have

The Ornish website[142] proclaims it the first program "scientifically proven to undo (reverse) heart disease." It refers to itself as "Intensive Cardiac Rehabilitation".

Proponents point to the diet as flexible and easy to follow, and some studies suggest that the Ornish Diet may help increase weight loss and protect against chronic disease. However being a strictly plant-based diet, it's also very low in healthy fats and may lack certain vitamins and minerals, so you need to monitor yourself for nutritional deficiencies.[143]

Detractors point to the lack of long-term studies and potentially statistically insignificant changes in cardiovascular health.[144]

Tobacco[145][146]

According to the CDC, tobacco use is the leading cause of preventable disease, disability, and death in the United States. Each year, nearly half a million Americans die prematurely of smoking or exposure to secondhand smoke, or about 1 in 5 deaths. Additionally, more than 16 million Americans live with a smoking-related disease. Each year, the United States spends more than $225 billion on medical care to treat smoking-related disease in adults.

Current smoking in U.S. adults has declined from 20.9% in 2005 to 12.5% in 2020. Unfortunately, this means that there are still an estimated 30.8 million adults in the United States currently smoking cigarettes, and an estimated 2.55 million middle and high school students use at least one tobacco product, including e-cigarettes. Every day, about 1,600 U.S. youth younger than 18 years smoke their first cigarette.

Bottom line, if you use tobacco, stop. There are many programs to help. Talk to your Primary Care Provider if you need assistance.

If you don't smoke, don't start.

Driving

Most crashes are caused by driver errors such as impaired driving, speeding, aggressive driving, or distracted driving. As a driver, you hold the key to crash prevention.[147]

- Share the Road (obey traffic laws)
- Don't drive impaired (Alcohol/drugs or tired)
- Drive Defensively
- Don't get Distracted (e.g., Cell Phone, Coffee, etc.)
- Wear Seatbelts

Detox your house[148]

HGTV shared 10 simple ideas to detox your house

- Don't wear shoes in your house to avoid bringing in pollutants
- Use Green Plants as Natural Detoxifiers
- Use wool dryer balls instead of dryer sheets
- Use cleaner cleaning products
- Add filters that remove fluoride, chemicals and heavy metals from your drinking water and showerhead

- Use a cotton shower curtain (vs PVC)
- Use a vacuum with a HEPA filter
- Eliminate as many plastics as you can
- Change out your mattresses to certified organic ones that are made by using no pesticides and manufactured by chemical-free processes
- If you have to dry clean take the bags off as soon as you get home then let them air out in a hall or garage for a couple of days to release some of the perchloroethylene solvents.

Personal Hygiene

Many hygiene-related diseases and conditions can be prevented or controlled by frequently washing parts of the body and hair with soap and clean, running water.[149]

Good personal hygiene is one of the best ways to protect yourself from getting gastro or infectious diseases (e.g., COVID-19, colds, and flu). Washing your hands with soap removes germs that can make you ill and will also help prevent you from spreading diseases to other people.[150]

Dental Health

You have millions of good and bad bacteria in your mouth called your oral microbiome. A balanced oral microbiome is crucial to your health. If there is negative imbalance in this microbiome, it can cause both oral and systemic diseases.[151] A negative imbalance in your oral microbiome can lead to:[152][153]

- Periodontal diseases
- Diseases of the digestive system (e.g., Inflammatory bowel syndrome)
- Cancer (oral, colorectal, and pancreatic cancer)
- Cardiovascular disease
- Alzheimers
- Diabetes
- Rheumatoid Arthritis

Below are some useful tips for keeping your oral microbiome healthy[154]

- Choose a "good bacteria"-boosting toothpaste
- Eat more plant-based foods
- Cut down on sugar
- Quit smoking
- If you are Diabetic, control your blood sugar

Health Benefits of Marriage

Married people appear to be healthier and live longer than those who are single, separated, divorced, or widowed. They have better mental health, fewer health conditions, and recover faster from illness.[155] Perhaps it is because healthy people are more likely to get married or it could be explained by the following:[156]

- Married people are more likely to have health insurance
- Having someone looking out for you and reinforcing healthy behaviors
- Marriage mitigates the health problems associated with loneliness and isolation

Get a Pet

Owning a pet comes with its own health benefits. Like little accountability partners, they can get us to exercise, get outside, and socialize more often. Additionally, pets through their companionship, can help manage loneliness and depression.[157] Man's best friend, indeed!

Bottom line, people with pets have:

- Higher survival rates
- Fewer heart attacks
- Less loneliness
- Better blood pressure
- Better cholesterol levels
- Better triglyceride levels
- Better psychological well-being
- Lower rates of depression and stress levels
- Fewer doctor visits
- Increased self-esteem
- Better sleep
- More physical activity

Get a Hobby

Hobbies can be very beneficial for our mental health. Studies have shown hobbies to give us lower stress, better physical health, more sleep, more social connections, improved work performance, and increased happiness.[158]

CHAPTER 9

HBOT AND OTHER THERAPIES

You know what they call alternative medicine that's been proved to work? Medicine.
~Tim Minchin

Hyperbaric Oxygen Therapy

Hyperbaric Oxygen Therapy (HBOT) is one of the most powerful, but most underutilized tools we have available.

How can hyperbaric therapy do what nothing else can do?

Let me say first, it does not cure everything. As a matter of fact, technically speaking, it does not cure anything. In the words of Dr. Jason Sonners in his excellent book **Oxygen Under Pressure (p. 119)**, "…hyperbaric therapy is instrumental in helping people with an enormously wide range of conditions, *but it does not treat disease (italics added)*. Oxygen is a required nutrient that, *when supplied in higher amounts(italics added)*, allows the body do what the body does: self-heal and self-regulate…to make cellular energy and heal itself."[159]

"HBOT is different than almost all of the other therapies we have. It is a biologic repair therapy, a foundation therapy upon which most other therapies can be added." (Dr. Paul G. Harch, MD in The Oxygen Revolution Third Edition p. 63)[160]

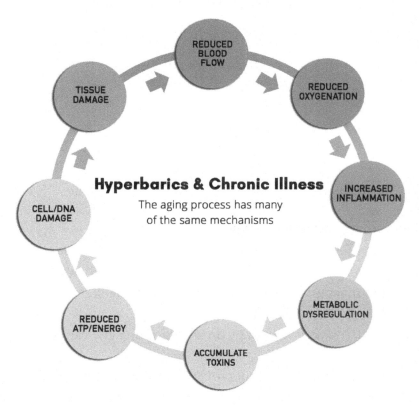

Hyperbarics & Chronic Illness
The Aging process shares many mechanisms with chronic illness.

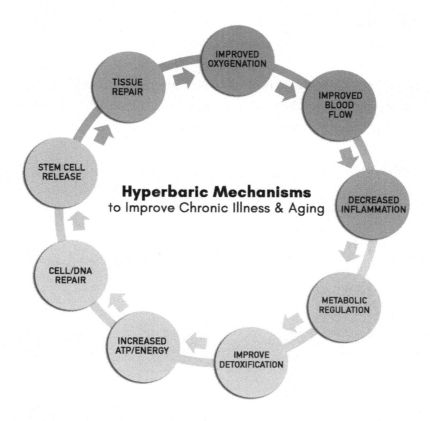

Hyperbaric Oxygen Mechanisms to Improve Chronic Illness and Aging

At its core, HBOT, or Hyperbaric Oxygen Therapy, is very simple. It adds oxygen to cells that need it. If the cell isn't working well, the oxygen helps to generate energy that promotes healing and removes toxins. This is an exciting new modality that can support healing in many tissues and conditions caused by inflammation, infections and wounds, musculoskeletal injuries, and neurodegenerative diseases. HBOT can also be used as a natural anti-aging and performance enhancer.[161] HBOT helps in these conditions because inflamed, injured tissue has impaired circulation and decreased oxygen perfusion. HBOT reverses these deficits and allows generation of the self-healing response; in other words, regeneration.

Hyperbaric Oxygen Therapy provides a multitude of benefits. There are approximately 100 conditions worldwide for which Hyperbaric Oxygen Therapy can be used to support healing, including:

Neurologic:

- Post-Stroke
- TBI/Concussion
- Chronic Fatigue
- Fibromyalgia
- ADD/ADHD
- Autism
- Cerebral Palsy
- Neuropathy

Neuro-Degenerative:

- Multiple sclerosis
- Parkinson's
- ALS
- Alzheimer's

Anti-aging/Performance:

- Memory loss
- Concussion
- Post exercise recovery
- Low energy
- Strains/sprains

Wounds/Infections:

- Lyme Disease
- Epstein Barr
- Post-surgical healing
- Scar healing

As of July 2021, there are 14 FDA Insurance approved Indications for Hyperbaric Oxygen Therapy:

- Air and gas bubbles in blood vessels
- Anemia (severe anemia when blood transfusions cannot be used)
- Burns (severe and large burns treated at a specialized burn center)
- Carbon monoxide poisoning
- Crush injury
- Decompression sickness (diving risk)
- Gas gangrene
- Hearing loss (complete hearing loss that occurs suddenly and without any known cause)
- Radiation injury
- Skin graft flap at risk of tissue death
- Vision loss (when sudden and painless in one eye due to blockage of blood flow)
- Non-healing, diabetic foot ulcers
- Infection of the skin and bone (severe)

There are over 100 International "off label" Indications for HBOT. Off label meaning it is not approved by the FDA, but has been used and found to support the body's natural healing response.

The power of HBOT is in the PRESSURE. By pressurizing oxygen, we are able to increase blood and tissue oxygen levels in areas where they are needed. Under these conditions, cellular energy is upregulated, promoting healing, peak performance, and optimal health and wellbeing. HBOT is a safe and effective way to restore, replenish and repair—a natural and highly effective therapeutic intervention.

Hyperbaric oxygen therapy, which involves breathing pure oxygen in a pressurized chamber, is often associated with high-profile professional athletes and celebrities looking to achieve peak performance and look and feel their best. Yet HBOT has actually been around for centuries, and has been used in this country for nearly 100 years to treat such conditions as decompression sickness, carbon monoxide poisoning, and diabetic foot ulcers and other wounds by delivering oxygen-rich plasma to our tissues and cells. HBOT works by pumping more oxygen into the body, stimulating the release of substances that promote healing.[162]

The more oxygen that goes into the body, the more it gets into the tissues and cells, initiating a host of healing responses. Our bodies really like oxygen.

In recent years, medical professionals have also been looking at hyperbaric oxygen therapy as a treatment for fatigue associated with long COVID, as well as a way to boost immunity to help prevent a host of diseases and improve overall quality of life.

Many NFL players have HBOT chambers in their homes to boost their performance, as well as recover from the normal wear and tear of the game. NFL and NBA players have HBOT chambers in their homes to boost their performance, as well as recover from the normal wear and tear of the game.

Steve Weatherford, NFL player:

"Despite how futuristic sleeping in hyperbaric chamber may seem, this has actually become a common practice among many NFL players for a few years now. I have my own portable chamber in my house! The reason for why I and so many NFL players engage in sleeping these chambers is because a hyperbaric chamber reduces swelling, promotes the healing of wounds, helps fight off dangerous infections, and increases the amount of oxygen in the bloodstream."[163]

After a serious injury in 2018, NBA superstar LeBron James used a hyperbaric oxygen chamber to aid in his recovery.[164] He and his personal trainer shared the story on Instagram and Twitter.

Additionally, it's a great way to prepare your body for surgery and heal your tissues after surgery or injury, reduce chronic inflammation, and so much more. HBOT supports the body's own natural healing process. When you do it over time, amazing things happen.

Mitochondria and Energy

One of the first benefits of HBOT is increased cellular energy. As oxygen is supplied to the cells, the mitochondria use this to create more ATP, the Energy molecule of the cell. As the mitochondria are exposed to oxygen repeatedly, damaged mitochondria heal and become more efficient. This helps provide the energy needed for metabolic regulation, healing and eventually tissue repair and regeneration.

Photobiomodulation, or Light Therapy

Photobiomodulation (PBM) describes the use of red or near-infrared light to stimulate, heal, regenerate, and protect tissue that has either been injured, is degenerating, or else is at risk of dying.[165] This can be either Low Level Laser Therapy, Infrared or Near-Infrared therapy. All these therapies transfer their energy to chromophores, molecules in the cells that absorb light. Certain wavelengths of light transfer energy that elicits healing.[166]

Infrared and Near Infrared Light[167]

Infrared therapy is a relatively new technique to treat pain and inflammation in various parts of the body. Unlike damaging ultraviolet light, infrared light is delivered to the site of injury or inflammation at certain wavelengths, promoting cell repair. Infrared light is safe, natural, non-invasive, and painless and can penetrate even the deep layers of the skin, therefore providing better pain relief.

Infrared therapy is widely used in the fields of medicine, dentistry, veterinary medicine, and in autoimmune diseases, to name a few. The therapy is offered as a safe and natural treatment for various health conditions supplementing medications and conventional treatments.

The risk of Infrared therapy are minimal. Thermal or heat injuries can happen, depending on the wavelength of the infrared light. Additionally, anyone who is pregnant, has heart disease, or is sick should avoid infrared therapy.

Low Level Laser Therapy[168]

Low Level Laser Therapy (LLLT) has benefits similar to Infrared and Near-Infrared Light. Lasers have higher energy output and can therefore penetrate deeper into tissue. LLLT has the same benefits as above, but in addition, the deeper penetration of light allows treatment of muscle, bone and joint issues.

Lasers are classified by their energy output, with Class 2 having the lowest energy but highest safety. Class 4 lasers have the highest energy. These are often called "medical grade lasers", meaning they are often used in medical settings for procedures.

Mitochondria and Light[169]

Mitochondria have light absorbing molecules, called chromophores. The chromophore in mitochondria is called cytochrome c. When we use specific wavelengths of light, energy in the light is transferred to cytochrome c, and it improves the energy output of the mitochondria. Providing this extra energy boosts the self-healing capabilities of the cells.

Light therapy has many roles in the human body. These include:[170]

- Detoxification
- Pain relief
- Reduction of muscle tension
- Relaxation
- Improved circulation
- Weight loss
- Skin lesions such as acne and herpes simplex

- Canker sores
- Lowered side effects of diabetes
- Boosting of the immune system
- Lowering of Blood Pressure

Chelation Therapy[171]

Chelation therapy was originally designed to treat metal poisoning. To date, this is the only FDA approved use for Chelation treatment. Since it's based on the process of chelation, in which chemicals are used to remove heavy metals and other substances from the body some health professionals have used chelation therapy for other ailments.

During Chelation therapy, a medication is injected which seeks out and sticks to metals and minerals in the bloodstream. This creates a compound that the body removes through normal renal-kidney function. Since it is thought that medicine will adhere to calcium in the arteries, Chelation therapy is promoted as a treatment for heart disease.[172]

In addition, chelation therapy is sometimes used to help support healing of the following health issues:

- Atherosclerosis (i.e., hardening of the arteries).
- Osteoarthritis and other inflammation-related conditions
- Autism
- Alzheimer's disease
- Band keratopathy
- Multiple sclerosis
- Peripheral artery disease

SECTION III:

WHAT VITALITY AND VIBRANCY CAN MEAN IN OUR LIVES

My mission in life is not merely to survive, but to thrive;
and to do so with some passion, some compassion, some humor,
and some style.
~Maya Angelou

There are five levels in Maslow's Hierarchy of Needs pyramid. From the bottom of the hierarchy upwards, the needs are: physiological (food and clothing), safety (job security), love and belonging needs (friendship), esteem, and self-actualization.[173]

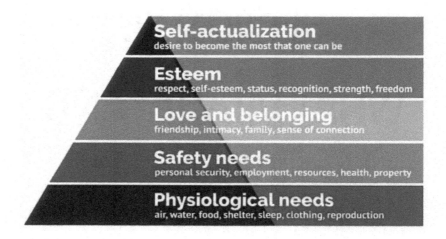

Now that we have covered air, water, food, sleep, and health, we are going to shift our focus to higher-level (Love and belonging, Esteem, and Self-Actualization) needs. Some of these topics already came up in Chapter 7 in the section on Mental Emotional Spiritual Health.

Namely, we need to find a way to work to live not live to work.

We need to have a reason to get up every day.

People either want more money, more time or more magic in their life. If money is not an issue, then magic in their lives becomes most important.
~Sean Callagy, Founder of Unblinded

*When we are speaking of magic in this context, we are not talking
about sleight of hand. We are talking about the real magic of
making a difference in the world.*
~Vincent Leonti, MD

Longevity. What exactly does that mean? Does that mean living
for as long as we can? When you ask people, many respond that
they don't want to live prolonged lives because of the ravages of
aging and infirmity, pain and suffering.

But, what if, you could live those years with vitality and viva-
ciousness? What if, you could live beyond 100 years and still be
able to enjoy family outings, play with the great great grandchildren, travel or whatever it is that would make you happy and
excited.

That is within reach for many of us. You only have to look at
what have been termed Blue Zones to see it is already happening. Blue Zones are communities where people routinely live
healthy vital lives into their 90s and even 100s. In his award-win-
ning books, Blue Zones and Blue Zones Challenge author Dan
Buettner details how these communities have lessons for all of
us: by building a foundation for better nutrition, more exercise,
and a stronger social life will extend your lifetime by years.

That is certainly a strong part of the foundation of what we
believe. Our hope is that his book can help extend those health
benefits and longevity to an even greater portion of the population, and create even more powerful benefits.

CHAPTER 10
CONTRIBUTION, IMPACT, LEGACY

It's not happy people who are thankful; it's thankful people who are happy.
~Unknown

Contribution

What you do makes a difference, and you have to decide what kind of difference you want to make.
~Jane Goodall

According to the Oxford Language Dictionary, Contribution is the part played by a person or thing in bringing about a result or helping something to advance.[174]

We contribute to make the world a better place all the time. The kindness we show, the smiles we give, the money we donate...all contribute to the well-being of the world. All these small steps are important and can bring joy to the world, and to us.

There is also contribution on a larger scale. Contribution with forethought, planning and execution that is meant to change the world in a meaningful, sustainable way for people or groups of people.

I have a vision that people do not die needlessly from preventable causes of death and that people do not suffer needlessly when help is available.

I started Princeton Integrative Health, along with my daughter, Jenna, and the support of my wife, Sue, with this vision in mind. As I progressed in my career in Emergency and then Family medicine, I found people who were ill and suffering, but I had no answers for them. The tools of conventional medicine, while great for the late stages of disease, are too blunt and rigid to deal with ills and suffering that do not fit its worldview.

When I opened my mind and heart and took my first course at the Institute of Functional Medicine, my whole Medical worldview changed. Functional and Integrative Medicine gave me a whole new set of tools to diagnose people's problems and to help relieve their suffering and eventually heal.

Helping create Princeton Integrative Health has been one of the joys of my life. On a daily basis, I can see examples of how we help to make people's lives better. Changing people's lives who come into direct contact with us is very fulfilling. But I consider that the first level of contribution.

Before I speak about the next level of contribution, we have to discuss another term: Impact.

Impact

There is no greater reward than working from your heart, and making a difference in the world.
~Carlos Santana

There are essentially two different, but interrelated impacts I want this book to make.

We cannot make impact unless we have the energy to do so.

I want this book to motivate people to take the health steps they need to maximize impact by creating vibrant energetic flow.

Then using this Energy, create a positive difference in the world.

The Impact Revolution is a movement in which we all play a part. It introduces a simple change, but one that has enormous ramifications for our world: the incorporation of impact - impact on our society and our environment - into the way we think, act and make decisions.
~Sir Ronald Cohen

Impact is:

"You can write a great book. But if only one person reads it, it's still a great book, but it doesn't have much impact." Ken Rochon, Dr. Smiley

That sums up impact as well as any definition I have read.

For greater impact, the next step is to educate and contribute to people we may never come into contact with. This book is an example of that. When I realized I had an important message, a message that could prevent suffering and save people's lives, I realized I had to write this book, to reach people who have not been reached before.

Energy/Flow

Many people think, if only I had more energy, I could accomplish that project or write that book. We often think, if I had more energy, I would go dance, or start exercising.

Have you ever noticed that some people seem to have endless energy? They seem to be able to get into the flow of whatever they are doing. Do you think they were born that way?

The good news is that while we may not all become super-achievers, we can all usually raise our energy. And that contributes to raising our mood.

How do we do this? One way is by physical movement, especially if it is fun such as dance. But, in a time crunch, just getting up and moving around, doing some jumping jacks if you can or some other higher intensity movement, can increase your energy and give you that boost for whatever it is you need to do.

For others, it's listening to music that is energizing or inspiring to them. Whether it is music or physical activity, both of these change our physiology and our brain activity. That's why they have the power to change our Energy and get us into the Flow.

Use your physical activity and music to change your brain.

Taking it to the Next Level

If this book motivates only one person to take action, to get checked and prevent a tragic, unnecessary death, then writing this book will be worth the effort. And if it can touch 100 or 1,000 or 1,000,000, then so much the better.

And if this book becomes part of a bigger movement to change the world for the better, not just for those we come into contact with, not just for those who read this book, but in joining forces with others to help change policy and change society so everyone can benefit. Everyone can benefit when it becomes the standard of care, part of the infrastructure of Medicine, the way things are done for everyone, not just those seeking it out. This is the Paradigm Shift in Medicine that we spoke about earlier in this book.

Contribution and Impact become a foundational part of *Your Personal Legacy.*

Legacy

> *Choose well. Your choice is brief, and yet endless.*
> ~Goethe

> *We all die. The goal isn't to live forever, it's to create something that will.*
> ~Chuck Palahniuk

From a purely practical standpoint, if you don't pass on your life experience by leaving a legacy, the wisdom you've gained through decades of difficult learning will disappear as your physical body wears out.
~Susan V. Bosak, Legacy Project Founder

A legacy may take many forms – children, grandchildren, a business, an ideal, a book, a community, a home, some piece of ourselves. Our legacy naturally intrigues us. It's perfectly understandable that we would want to know how the world will remember us after we're gone. How many of us will be surprised? How many of us are living our lives so that our legacy reflects all that we truly hold most near and dear? How many of us are living with integrity and courage?

Most of us do the best we can. And that's all anyone can ask. The Legacy Project[175] is about helping you do the very best you can. (https://www.legacyproject.org/guides/whatislegacy.html)

When you define and create your Contribution and multiply its effect through maximizing Impact, you are doing as Susan V. Bosak exhorts above, to **"do the very best you can."**

For me, ultimately, I would like for my contribution to be a healthier world, where people have more control over their health and treatment and live longer, happier, more fulfilled lives. We know health impacts have multi-generational consequences. Poor diet, smoking and other unhealthy behaviors can have negative consequences on succeeding generations. I want to help people create health and health behaviors with positive multi-generational impacts. Instead of a multi-generational vicious cycle, let's start a multi-generational Virtuous Cycle of improving health with every generation. No time is more important than now, when we have seen decreases in Life Expectancy even pre-COVID.

What do you want your Legacy to be? Stay tuned as we create an Interactive Page to discuss this and other topics in Staying Alive.

APPENDiX A: ACTION STEPS

- Go dancing. Don't know how to dance, take a dance class
- Play checkers with a young person. Play checkers with an old person. Play checkers with someone in between
- Go for a Hike
- Play Pickleball. Don't know how, take a class
- Relax
- Read a book
- Learn something new
- Teach someone something new.
- Take a cooking class...Teach a cooking class
- Collect memories not things
- Create a Bucket List...Work daily towards completing it
- Travel
  - Meet a friend for lunch. Even if you don't need it, they may
- You have a lifetime of wisdom, share it
- Save the next generation from making the same mistakes you did

- Share your family lore
- Preserve culture and traditions and create a link to the past
- Record it / write it down
- Create a Cookbook of Family recipes
- Do something every day to challenge you and sharpen your mind (there are now Apps on your phone for all of these)
- Crossword Puzzles
  - Sudoku
  - Solitaire
- Volunteer
  - Library
  - School
  - Shelter
  - Hospital

APPENDIX B: QUICK START GUIDE[176]

Home electronics once came with a detailed instruction manual that most people ignored until they had a problem. Now they come with a Quick Start Guide, which are basic procedures on what you need to get started.

Consider this your Quick Start Guide.

Items to be discussed with you doctor for assessment include:

1. Insulin Resistance
    __Fasting Glucose (included on Comprehensive Metabolic Panel)
    __Fasting Insulin

2. Inflammatory Markers in Blood and Urine
    __Myeloperoxidase
    __Lp-PLA-2
    __hs-CRP

__ADMA/SDMA
__oxidized LDL
__Microalbumin Creatinine ratio Urine
__F2-Isoprostanes Urine

3. Genetic Markers:
   __ApoE
   __9p21
   __Lipoprotein-a
   Other Bloodwork
   __Lipid panel with Lipoprotein fractionation:
   __Thyroid Panel
   __Vitamin D, Folate and B12
   __Ferritin: Iron storage hormone
   __Iron with Total Iron Binding Capacity(TIBC)
   __CMP (Comprehensive Metabolic Panel)
   __CBC (Complete Blood Count)

4. Sleep Testing
   __Overnight Oximetry
   __Home Sleep Test
   __Hospital Sleep Test

5. __EKG

6. CIMT and Coronary Calcium Scoring
   __CIMT (Carotid Intima Media Thickness) Ultrasound
   __Coronary Calcium Scoring

7. Oral Health
   __My Periopath from Oral DNA Labs

APPENDIX C: EXPLANATIONS FOR THE QUICK START GUIDE

1. Insulin Resistance:

Do you have Insulin Resistance?

For the vast majority of people with Insulin Resistance, it is straightforward to diagnose.

Bloodwork to be done:

___Fasting Glucose

___Fasting Insulin

___Calculate HOMA-IR* (HIR) (Glucose (mg/dl) xInsulin (uIu/ml))/400=HIR

HIR less than 1: Optimal Insulin Sensitivity

HIR 1.1 to 1.9: You could be developing Insulin Resistance

HIR 2.0 to 2.9 correlates with early Insulin Resistance

HIR 3.0 or above correlates with significant Insulin Resistance

Examples:

A. Fasting Glucose 85. Insulin 4. (85x4)/400= 340/400=0.85. This is less than 1, thus optimal Insulin Sensitivity

B. Fasting Glucose: 95 Fasting Insulin 7: (95x7)/400=665/400=1.66. Between 1 and 2, could be developing Insulin Resistance. Further assessment needed.

C. Fasting Glucose: 95 Fasting Insulin 10: (95x10)/400=950/400=2.38. over 2, less than 3, early Insulin Resistance.

D. Fasting Glucose: 95 Fasting Insulin 15: (95x15)/400=1425/400=3.56. over 3, significant Insulin Resistance.

Occasionally people may need more advanced testing such as a 2 hr oral Glucose Tolerance test to diagnose Insulin Resistance.

2. **Bloodwork that includes the following Inflammatory markers:**

Myeloperoxidase: Marker of Blood Vessel and Plaque Inflammation

Lp-PLA2 (Lipoprotein Associated Phospholipase A2): Marker of Blood Vessel and Plaque Inflammation

hs-CRP (high sensitivity C-reactive protein)—marker of systemic inflammation

ADMA/SDMA—tells us about the health of the endothelium and its ability to produce Nitric Oxide.

oxLDL (oxidized LDL): The inflamed portion of the LDL

MACR (Urine Microalbumin/Creatinine Ratio): Evaluates albumin in the urine. This tells us about the health of the Endothelium and whether it is leaky, leaking albumin into the Urine. A leaky Endothelium is a strong risk factor for Vascular Inflammation

F2-Isoprostanes/Creatinine Ratio (Urine): Tells us about oxidative stress in the body

3. Genetic markers:

ApoE: Receive 1 copy of each gene designated as 2,3 or 4. If you have 1 or 2 copies of the 4 variant, your body reacts with more inflammation.

9p21: The so-called Heart Attack gene. This gene confers a higher risk of developing heart disease, especially with poor diet.

Lp(a) (Lipoprotein (a)): An inherited Lipoprotein disorder. Affects 20% of the population. Not included in standard cholesterol panels.

The importance of knowing your genetic markers is that, their risk is modifiable. If you have one or more of these genetic markers, we know you and your risk factors need to be treated more intensely.

4. **Other bloodwork that can be helpful:**

Lipid panel with Lipoprotein fractionation: a deeper look at cholesterol risk

Thyroid Panel: Affects metabolism, including Cholesterol

Vitamin D, Folate and B12: Affects Heart, vascular, glucose regulation and nerve health

Ferritin: Iron storage hormone. Can indicate Inflammation

Iron with Total Iron Binding Capacity(TIBC): Serum Iron and TIBC

CMP (Comprehensive Metabolic Panel)

CBC (Complete Blood Count)

5. **Sleep Testing**

Sleep apnea is still an underdiagnosed risk factor.

Should have at the minimum an overnight oximetry (oxygen monitoring) test.

Home Sleep Tests are a better option because they give more information.

In hospital sleep tests are the most comprehensive option.

6. **EKG:** Looks at the electrical activity of the heart. Good to have as a baseline so changes can be more easily detected.

7. **CIMT and Coronary Calcium Scoring**

CIMT(Carotid Intima Media Thickness): This Non-invasive Vascular Ultrasound gives us information about Plaque and Inflammation in the Blood Vessel Wall. 80% correlation with the status of the Coronary Arteries. This testing allows us to better determine risk and treatment strategies. The power of this test is also that you can follow this every 9 to 12 months and see changes in the Carotid Arteries. This can tell us whether treatment strategies are working to improve the health of the arteries. And that is the whole point of everything we are doing: Improve the health of the Arteries to prevent Heart Attack, and Dementia.

Coronary Calcium scoring can see calcified plaque in the Coronary Arteries, indicating Coronary Artery Disease. You get a dose of Ionizing Radiation with this test. Not everyone needs it, and due to the radiation, it should not be a test done frequently.

8. **Oral Health: Microbiome Testing and Gum Disease**

Gum Health and Microbiome are intimately connected to Systemic Health.

Oral bacteria have been found in the brains of Alzheimer's patients and at the site of plaque rupture of heart attack victims. You can see how important Oral Health is.

If you have any bleeding with brushing or flossing or during dental cleanings, that is definitely abnormal and a sign of gum disease.

If your gum pockets are over 3 mm depth, that is a sign of gum disease.

Do a Salivary Diagnostic Test called My Periopath from Oral DNA Labs. This will inform whether you have High Risk Bacteria in your mouth. High Risk bacteria means bacteria which are more likely to penetrate into the bloodstream and cause systemic disease.

If you have any of the above, you will need a dentist or periodontist to do a deep cleaning and treatment to take care of the issues.

BIOGRAPHY

Dr. Vincent Leonti, MD
Medical Director

Dr. Leonti knew from the time he was in grade school that he wanted to become a doctor. After graduating from SUNY Upstate Medical University in Syracuse, NY, he went back and forth between family medicine and emergency medicine. His preference was for family medicine because it allowed him to develop closer relationships with his patients.

Dr. Leonti has always been active. He has even completed five marathons over the years. That's why he was shocked when he went out for a run one day and experienced pain in his chest. A cardiologist told Dr. Leonti that he had an 80 percent blockage in one coronary artery and a 70 percent blockage in another.

As a doctor, Dr. Leonti thought he was living a healthy lifestyle, but he unknowingly had been misinformed and developed bad habits that brought him to an unhealthy place. He was forced to make lifestyle changes to improve his health. It was during this time that his daughter, Jenna, began her journey in functional medicine and integrative health.

Dr. Leonti had never heard of functional medicine and admittedly thought the concept was more than a little off-base. It seemed to go against everything he knew as a medical doctor. He skeptically attended his first functional medicine conference and instantly saw the disconnect between traditional and functional medicine. Traditional medicine was great at treating acute illness or crisis situations, like a broken arm or heart attack, but chronic illness was a different story.

Dr. Leonti realized that so much more could be done to prevent and reverse chronic illness by bringing the functional approach to conventional medicine. Instead of waiting for a problem to arise and treating it with medication, functional medicine attacks the root cause of health issues and prevents problems from occurring in the first place. Dr. Leonti enrolled in the Institute for Functional Medicine and Functional Medicine University, where he is in process of certification.

The real-life experiences of a father and daughter, and a shared belief in the power of functional and conventional medicine, soon led to the creation of Princeton Integrative Health.

INDEX

addiction, 104

alcohol, 29, 31, 36, 43, 51, 57, 62, 80, 93, 95, 99, 104, 106, 113

Anemia, 72, 121

anxiety, 30, 93, 95-96, 108

asthma, 100

blood pressure, xii, 4, 29-30, 35, 53, 55, 57-58, 65, 73, 76, 80, 87, 92, 96, 99-100, 116, 126

blood sugar, 6, 30, 34, 44, 47-50, 58, 60, 79, 101, 115

caffeine, 79, 95

Calcium, 7, 55, 69-70, 73-74, 126, 142, 147

cancer, x, 26-30, 50, 52-53, 70-71, 73, 75, 80, 115

carbohydrate, 50, 59, 68

Cardiac Disease, x, 87

cholesterol, 4, 6, 27, 29, 33, 50, 53, 57-58, 76, 101, 116, 145-146

chronic pain, 95-96, 108

COVID, viii, ix, 12, 20, 35, 71-72, 93, 122

death, x, 4, 9, 12-13, 22, 26-30, 58, 67, 76, 80, 92, 100, 104, 112, 121, 132, 135

dementia, x, 11, 28-30, 35, 53, 147

depression, 8-9, 26, 30, 92, 95-97, 108-109, 116

Detox, iii, vi, 41, 56, 63-64, 113

diabetes, xi, 9, 22, 27, 29-30, 42, 47-48, 50, 52-54, 59, 61, 65, 71-72, 81, 83, 92, 99-100, 115, 126, 157

diabetic, 48, 115, 121-122

diet, iii, vi, vii, x, 4, 6, 9, 23, 29, 35, 37, 40-42, 44-45, 47-49, 51-61, 66, 68-69, 73-74, 77, 81, 83, 94, 106, 111-112, 136, 145

drugs, xii, 21, 62, 93, 104, 113

energy, x, 2, 12-13, 52-53, 76, 79, 81, 88, 92, 108-109, 118-120, 122-125, 133-134

exercise, iii, 2, 6, 20, 23, 26, 30, 40, 42, 59, 85, 87-88, 95, 105-106, 116, 120, 129

fat, 9, 47, 50-52, 58-59, 64-65, 68, 82, 111

fatigue, 12, 79, 100, 108, 120, 122

fatty liver, 81-82, 101

fiber, 49-51, 55, 62

Graded Exercise, 87

heart attack, xi, 4, 6-7, 10, 13, 35, 87, 100, 145, 147-148, 150

heart disease, vii, viii, ix, xi, xii, 4, 6-7, 9-13, 22-23, 25, 28-30, 33, 42, 50, 54, 58, 65, 71, 76, 81, 92, 100-101, 112, 124, 126, 145

high blood pressure, xii, 29, 35, 80, 92, 99-100

hormones, 34, 66, 76, 84

hypertension, 42, 58

Immune System, 37-38, 76, 126

immunity, 37, 122

infection, 21, 37, 121

inflammation, 11, 22, 33, 35, 38, 49, 61, 67, 69-70, 76, 108, 119, 123-124, 144-147

inflammatory bowel disease, 61, 65

Insulin, 9, 22, 33-34, 44, 47-48, 52-53, 57, 59, 81-82, 93, 100, 141, 143-144

Insulin Resistance, 9, 22, 33-34, 44, 47, 53, 59, 81-82, 93, 100, 141, 143-144

Insulin Sensitivity, 53, 144

Leaky Gut, 61, 67

Memory, xi, 65, 105, 120

Mental Health, x, 23, 34, 40, 85, 88, 92-93, 95, 103-104, 115-116

obesity, 9, 27, 29, 31, 42, 51, 53-54, 65, 81, 83-84, 92

oxidative stress, 47, 145

pain, 1, 5, 7, 61, 75, 86, 95-96, 100, 108, 124-125, 129, 149

Parkinson Disease, —

pre-diabetes, 27, 47, 50, 59

protein, 43-44, 49, 52, 55, 57-60, 68, 70, 74, 145

Rheumatoid Arthritis, 61, 115

sleep, iii, 2, 23, 27, 30, 33-35, 37, 40, 79, 85, 91-101, 105-106, 108, 116, 128, 142, 146-147

sleep apnea, 33, 35, 98-101, 146

smoking, 23, 26, 29-31, 33, 59, 99, 112, 115, 136

stress, iii, 2, 7-8, 34-35, 37, 47, 85, 87-88, 92-94, 103-106, 108-109, 111, 116, 145

stress test, 7-8, 35, 87

stroke, x, xi, 6, 10, 23, 25, 28-29, 35, 92, 100

sugar, 6, 30, 34, 37, 44, 47-50, 55, 57-58, 60, 68, 79, 81-83, 101, 115

supplements, iii, vi, xii, 37-38, 41, 50-51, 56, 58, 64, 68-70, 73-74, 76-77, 96-97

tobacco, 26, 29, 62, 95, 106, 112-113

toxins, 63-64, 119

water, 45, 51, 56, 64, 78-79, 108, 113-114, 128

REFERENCES

1   https://www.heart.org/en/get-involved/advocate/
    federal-priorities/cdc-prevention-programs
2   (https://www.globenewswire.com/fr/
    news-release/2021/09/23/2301830/0/en/Helen-Keller-s-
    Vision-for-the-Future-Disrupts-Traditional-Fundraising-
    for-the-American-Foundation-for-the-Blind-AFB.html)
3   https://www.managedhealthcareexecutive.com/view/
    the-u-s-healthcare-system-is-broken-a-national-perspective
4   https://www.health.harvard.edu/blog/
    is-our-healthcare-system-broken-202107132542
5   https://www.who.int/news-room/facts-in-pictures/detail/
    diabetes
6   https://www.cdc.gov/nchs/data/hus/2019/006-508.pdf
7   https://pubmed.ncbi.nlm.nih.gov/23435157/
8   https://www.heart.org/en/get-involved/advocate/
    federal-priorities/cdc-prevention-programs
9   https://newsroom.clevelandclinic.org/2021/09/29/90-per-
    cent-of-heart-disease-is-preventable-through-healthier-
    diet-regular-exercise-and-not-smoking/#:~:text=2021%20
    %2F%20News%20Updates-,90%20Percent%20of%20
    Heart%20Disease%20is%20Preventable%20through%20

Healthier%20Diet,regular%20exercise%2C%20and%20
not%20smoking

10   https://www.ahajournals.org/doi/10.1161/
CIR.0000000000001052

11   https://www.cdc.gov/tobacco/campaign/tips/
resources/data/cigarette-smoking-in-united-states.
html?s_cid=OSH_tips_GL0005&utm_source=-
google&utm_medium=cpc&utm_campaign=TipsRegu-
lar+2021%3BS%3BWL%3BBR%3BIMM%3BDTC%3B-
CO&utm_content=Smoking+-+Facts_P&utm_term=infor-
mation+about+smoking&gclid=Cj0KCQjwm6KUBhC3A-
RIsACIwxBi8DzYt1yDmP_w2UOzfSU7raGX3uBj3Mvn-
PoyiML2H6WNrQ5OqtYvIaAhmgEALw_wcB&gclsrc=aw.
ds

12   https://www.cdc.gov/nchs/products/databriefs/db427.htm

13   https://www.americashealthrankings.org/explore/annual/
measure/YPLL/state/ALL

14   https://www.prb.org/resources/up-to-half-of-u-s-prema-
ture-deaths-are-preventable-behavioral-factors-key/#:~:-
text=Four%20factors%E2%80%94poor%20diet%2C%20
high,of%20the%20University%20of%20Washington.

15   https://theconversation.com/obesity-second-to-smoking-
as-the-most-preventable-cause-of-us-deaths-needs-new-ap-
proaches-129317

16   https://www.niaaa.nih.gov/publi-
cations/brochures-and-fact-sheets/
understanding-alcohol-impact-health

17   https://www.cdc.gov/vitalsigns/heartdisease-stroke/

18   https://www.cdc.gov/aging/publications/features/demen-
tia-not-normal-aging.html

19   https://www.cdc.gov/chronicdisease/resources/publications/
factsheets/cancer.htm

20   https://www.aha.org/news/headline/2022-05-12-aha-ama-ana-mark-grim-milestone-us-covid-19-deaths-surpass-1-million

21   https://l.facebook.com/l.php?u=https%3A%2F%2Fvimeo.com%2F399733860%3Ffbclid%3DIwAR1-RPAeWJQ-cav6u7cZYFfWCZ2xNy5te5xDa5HelgAEQ6kp3RAVk-Sh2rWP8&h=AT1bh4MRCFeXIrAgC5I_gvTEKHsGZ-yp4-wxPDpDACWujPjza7S0-lCrNoBINlV9HDgiCxfT-NVsJwKnYHTGfjAeu-dXEK6trj9h4GO3A0onrxy1wRr_X9pvnviAAWUoWpZ4aGr4q-7B1J8mA

22   https://vimeo.com/399733860?fbclid=IwAR2a7p-qZ5_k1Gn0yogIedJUBLRdBQotA3XIZuGlR3elheHDUrehHqH-HJFc

23   https://www.facebook.com/princetonintegrativehealth/photos/a.1762268787430764/3279393139051647/?type=3

24   https://www.ncbi.nlm.nih.gov/books/NBK499830/

25   https://www.heart.org/en/healthy-living/healthy-eating/eat-smart/nutrition-basics/aha-diet-and-lifestyle-recommendations

26   ChooseMyPlate.gov

27   https://www.disabled-world.com/fitness/nutrition/myplate.php

28   https://baumancollege.org/eating-for-health/

29   https://baumancollege.org/eating-for-health/

30   Fung, J. (2018). The Diabetes Code, Prevent and Reverse Type 2 Diabetes Naturally. Greystone Books Ltd.

31   https://www.cdc.gov/diabetes/library/features/role-of-fiber.html

32   https://www.webmd.com/vitamins-and-supplements/supplement-guide-fiber

33   https://www.cdc.gov/diabetes/library/features/role-of-fiber.html

34 https://www.ncbi.nlm.nih.gov/pmc/articles/PMC6466433/

35 https://www.ncbi.nlm.nih.gov/books/NBK499830/

36 https://www.mayoclinic.org/healthy-lifestyle/nutri-tion-and-healthy-eating/in-depth/paleo-diet/art-20111182

37 https://news.llu.edu/patient-care/beginner-s-guide-dan-iel-fast-diet#:~:text=The%20Daniel%20Fast%20diet%20consists,legumes%2C%20nuts%2C%20and%20seeds

38 https://www.healthline.com/nutrition/daniel-diet#basics

39 https://www.healthline.com/nutrition/daniel-diet#food-lists

40 https://www.ncbi.nlm.nih.gov/pmc/articles/PMC2941756/

41 https://www.health.harvard.edu/blog/plant-based-diets-are-best-or-are-they-2019103118122

42 https://www.pcrm.org/news/blog/cdc-should-prescribe-plant-based-diet-middle-aged-hearts

43 https://theconversation.com/why-people-become-veg-ans-the-history-sex-and-science-of-a-meatless-existence-106410#:~:text=Like%20other%20alternative%20food%20movements,and%20better%20for%20the%20environment.

44 https://www.ncbi.nlm.nih.gov/pmc/articles/PMC3662288/

45 https://chriskresser.com/do-vegetarians-and-vegans-live-longer-than-meat-eaters/

46 https://www.additudemag.com/adhd-diet-nutrition-sugar/

47 https://www.healthline.com/nutrition/aip-diet-autoimmune-protocol-diet

48 https://l.facebook.com/l.php?u=https%3A%2F%2Fwww.ncbi.nlm.nih.gov%2Fpmc%2Farticles%2FPMC6592837%2F%3Ff-bclid%3DIwAR11X7FIOLo0FK0QoZ2gF9QzABJi-3y7vK6nyBUVdXQ1P_ALaMTvWbfmWjYc&h=AT1x_e_IA8yFACOnmKOPnjS6h5bR7PAl3l0vOxi2jo5T4qQT_bBzDAe2aOwP9FcZLypy_zreMlsiIYY-

iog8xbcx1juOWSYolsvwU9TYrDGWoQ_
Eu3pW6M7BOQGly4yrOMuCOhY8r8kWHRyDch461&__
tn__=%2CmH-R&c[0]=AT0ieVVVvmfrbRwGBVHCB-
HOCtDQZnNaoJnKaR_djWKgcRvRrN1H7Zm55scm-
BiKmh2sub9YJ9EP6BQUM5gR7rmp_5uEKtm6nd-
cPTjiXfq7sLi7H8Vq4JhxKziILd_yH1rv8AKAGW5gBvleY-
I9grMF40Suk0hXWHtbTT4_L1qjATkLvTE

49 https://www.nccih.nih.gov/health/
    detoxes-and-cleanses-what-you-need-to-know

50 https://www.naturallynourishedrd.com/5-reasons-you-
    need-to-detox-and-keeping-your-keto-clean/

51 https://www.hopkinsmedicine.org/
    health/wellness-and-prevention/
    intermittent-fasting-what-is-it-and-how-does-it-work

52 https://www.heart.org/en/healthy-living/healthy-eating/
    eat-smart/nutrition-basics/organic-food-fact-vs-percep-
    tion#:~:text=AHA%20encourages%20consumers%20to%20
    eat,and%20fiber%20for%20healthy%20diets.

53 https://www.ewg.org/foodnews/dirty-dozen.php

54 https://www.amymyersmd.com/article/
    avoid-gmos-autoimmune-disease/

55 https://www.insider.com/gmo-pros-and-cons

56 https://www.amymyersmd.com/article/
    avoid-gmos-autoimmune-disease/

57 https://www.hsph.harvard.edu/nutritionsource/vita-
    min-d/#:~:text=Also%2C%20laboratory%20studies%20
    show%20that,actively%20investigating%20other%20
    possible%20functions.

58 https://www.mayoclinic.org/drugs-supplements-vitamin-d/
    art-20363792

59 https://www.jabfm.org/content/22/6/698

60 https://www.hsph.harvard.edu/nutritionsource/vita-min-d/#:~:text=Also%2C%20laboratory%20studies%20show%20that,actively%20investigating%20other%20possible%20functions.

61 https://pubmed.ncbi.nlm.nih.gov/34607398/

62 Holick MF, Binkley NC, Bischoff-Ferrari HA, et al. Evaluation, treatment, and prevention of vitamin D deficiency: An Endocrine Society clinical practice guideline. Journal of Clinical Endocrinology & Metabolism 2011

63 Heaney RP, Holick MF. Why the IOM recommendations for vitamin D are deficient. Journal of Bone and Mineral Research

64 https://www.webmd.com/diet/features/the-benefits-of-vita-min-c#:~:text=Vitamin%20C%2C%20also%20known%20as,cartilage%2C%20bones%2C%20and%20teeth.

65 https://www.medicalnewstoday.com/articles/219352#other-benefits

66 https://www.medicalnewstoday.com/articles/219352#requirements

67 https://www.mayoclinic.org/drugs-supplements-vitamin-c/art-20363932

68 https://www.hsph.harvard.edu/nutritionsource/cal-cium/#:~:text=Calcium%20is%20a%20mineral%20most,heart%20rhythms%20and%20nerve%20functions.

69 https://www.orthoillinois.com/blog/12-things-you-need-to-know-about-calcium-supplements-for-bone-health/

70 https://www.frieslandcampinainstitute.com/ng/dairy/milk/calcium-supplement-good-alternative-drinking-milk/

71 {https://www.ncbi.nlm.nih.gov/pmc/articles/PMC5786912/}

72 https://www.healthline.com/nutrition/turmeric-dosage#benefits

73 https://www.medicalnewstoday.com/articles/318405#benefits

74   https://ods.od.nih.gov/factsheets/Omega3FattyAcids-
     Consumer/#:~:text=Omega%2D3%20fatty%20acids%20
     are,%2C%20soybean%2C%20and%20canola%20oils.

75   https://www.hsph.harvard.edu/nutritionsource/what-should-
     you-eat/fats-and-cholesterol/types-of-fat/omega-3-fats/

76   https://my.clevelandclinic.org/health/
     articles/17290-omega-3-fatty-acids

77   https://www.zmescience.com/other/feature-post/
     how-long-survive-no-food-water-052352/

78   https://www.timesnownews.com/health/article/
     hydration-tips-is-there-a-correct-way-to-drink-water-all-
     you-need-to-know/633188

79   https://www.mayoclinic.org/healthy-lifestyle/
     nutrition-and-healthy-eating/in-depth/water/
     art-20044256#:~:text=The%20U.S.%20National%20
     Academies%20of,fluids%20a%20day%20for%20women

80   https://www.cdc.gov/niosh/emres/longhourstraining/
     caffeine.html

81   https://www.cdc.gov/niosh/emres/longhourstraining/
     caffeine.html

82   https://www.cdc.gov/niosh/emres/longhourstraining/using-
     caffeine.html

83   https://www.fda.gov/consumers/consumer-updates/spill-
     ing-beans-how-much-caffeine-too-much#:~:text=For%20
     healthy%20adults%2C%20the%20FDA,associated%20
     with%20dangerous%2C%20negative%20effects.

84   https://www.cdc.gov/niosh/emres/longhourstraining/using-
     caffeine.html

85   https://www.addictioncenter.com/alcohol/is-alcohol-a-de-
     pressant/#:~:text=Alcohol%20can%20depress%20the%20
     central,lessens%20inhibitions%2C%20and%20distorts%20
     judgment.

86   https://www.cdc.gov/alcohol/fact-sheets/moderate-drinking.html
87   https://www.dietaryguidelines.gov/resources/2020-2025-dietary-guidelines-online-materials
88   https://www.cdc.gov/nutrition/data-statistics/sugar-sweetened-beverages-intake.html
89   https://www.healthline.com/nutrition/foods-with-high-fructose-corn-syrup
90   https://www.pennmedicine.org/news/news-releases/2020/june/the-gut-shields-the-liver-from-fructose-induced-damage#:~:text=When%20large%20quantities%20of%20fructose,stored%20in%20the%20liver%20cells.
91   https://health.clevelandclinic.org/what-is-fructose-intolerance/
92   https://blog.thefastingmethod.com/the-diet-soda-delusion-the-epiphenomenon-of-obesity-5/
93   https://www.health.harvard.edu/staying-healthy/is-plastic-a-threat-to-your-health#:~:text=Studies%20have%20found%20that%20certain,including%20obesity)%20and%20reduced%20fertility.
94   https://sportscardiologybc.org/stretching-the-hidden-benefits-to-health-and-fitness/
95   https://cooperaerobics.com/Health-Tips/Fitness-Files/Top-Five-Aerobic-Activities.aspx
96   https://www.healthline.com/health/fitness-exercise/anaerobic-exercise
97   https://www.stretchzone.com/blog-posts/table-stretching-forms/#:~:text=There%20are%20four%20types%20of,stretching%2C%20which%20involves%20table%20stretching.
98   https://trilliumhealthpartners.ca/patientservices/cardiacservices/cardiopulmonaryservices/cardiacdiagnostics/Pages/

Graded-Exercise-Stress-TestingMetabolic-Exercise-Stress-Testing.aspx

99 https://www.unitypoint.org/livewell/article.aspx?id=711c3612-4a77-45d6-996b-d2ae51416a75

100 https://www.ncbi.nlm.nih.gov/pmc/articles/PMC2014801/#:~:text=These%20stress%20tests%2C%20usually%20called,beats%20per%20minute%20(4).

101 https://www.hindawi.com/journals/ecam/2017/8763915/

102 https://www.cancer.gov/publications/dictionaries/cancer-terms/def/mind-body-exercise#:~:text=Listen%20to%20pronunciation,%2C%20tai%20chi%2C%20and%20qigong.

103 https://www.physio-pedia.com/Parasympathetic_System

104 https://www.sleepfoundation.org/how-sleep-works/why-do-we-need-sleep#:~:text=Sleep%20is%20an%20essential%20function,the%20brain%20cannot%20function%20properly.

105 https://www.cdc.gov/sleep/index.html

106 https://niach.ernesthealth.com/how-sleep-helps-healing/#:~:text=Restful%20sleep%20cycles%20are%20imperative,tissue%2C%20bone%2C%20and%20muscle.

107 https://www.chicagotribune.com/suburbs/advertising/marketplace/ct-ss-suburbs-four-crucial-ways-that-sleep-helps-the-body-to-heal-20180112dto-story.html

108 https://www.sleepfoundation.org/how-sleep-works/why-do-we-need-sleep#:~:text=Sleep%20is%20an%20essential%20function,the%20brain%20cannot%20function%20properly.

109 https://www.ncbi.nlm.nih.gov/pmc/articles/PMC4589931/

110 https://www.sleepfoundation.org/physical-health/pain-and-sleep

111 https://www.sciencedirect.com/science/article/abs/pii/S0022399917308486

112 https://www.hopkinsmedicine.org/
health/wellness-and-prevention/
depression-and-sleep-understanding-the-connection

113 https://www.sciencedirect.com/science/article/abs/pii/
S0022399917308486

114 https://www.nccih.nih.gov/health/
melatonin-what-you-need-to-know

115 https://www.healthline.com/nutrition/melatonin

116 https://www.hopkinsmedicine.org/health/
wellness-and-prevention/melatonin-for-sleep-does-it-work

117 https://www.sleepfoundation.org/sleep-aids/
how-to-use-sleep-medications-safely

118 https://www.medicinenet.com/are_sleeping_pills_bad_for_
you/article.htm#:~:text=Some%20sleeping%20pills%20
may%20cause,use%20sleeping%20pills%20every%20night

119 https://www.thensf.org/

120 https://www.thensf.org/national-sleep-foundation-an-
nounces-sleep-awareness-week-2022-dates/#:~:text=Wash-
ington%2C%20D.C.%20(February%2018%2C,measure%20
of%20their%20overall%20health.

121 https://www.thensf.org/drowsy-driving-prevention/

122 https://www.mayoclinic.org/diseases-conditions/
sleep-apnea/symptoms-causes/syc-20377631

123 https://people.com/country/naomi-judd-dead-at-76/

124 https://wisqars.cdc.gov/data/lcd/home

125 https://www.cdc.gov/nchs/fastats/leading-causes-of-death.
htm

126 https://screening.mhanational.org/screening-tools/

127 https://www.cdc.gov/mentalhealth/learn/index.htm

128 https://www.betterup.com/blog/emotional-health-examples

129 https://www.webmd.com/balance/
how-spirituality-affects-mental-health

130 https://greatergood.berkeley.edu/article/item/
the_surprising_benefits_of_stress

131 https://www.webmd.com/balance/guide/all-stressed-out-
#:~:text=On%20the%20other%20hand%2C%20
negative,%2C%20health%20problems%2C%20and%20
exhaustion.

132 https://health.gov/myhealthfinder/topics/health-conditions/
heart-health/manage-stress

133 https://www.cdc.gov/violenceprevention/about/coping-
with-stresstips.html

134 https://www.facebook.com/princetonintegrativehealth/
photos/a.1762268787430764/3285993588391602/?type=3

135 https://globalwellnessinstitute.org/wellnessevidence/
forest-bathing/

136 https://www.healthline.com/health/grounding#:~:tex-
t=Grounding%2C%20also%20called%20earthing%2C%20
is,positive%20effects%20on%20your%20body.

137 https://www.sciencedirect.com/science/article/pii/
S1550830719305476

138 https://www.ncbi.nlm.nih.gov/pmc/articles/PMC4378297/

139 https://pubmed.ncbi.nlm.nih.gov/30448083/

140 https://www.haymsalomonhome.com/
four-health-benefits-of-fun/

141 https://www.medpagetoday.com/opinion/skepti-
cal-cardiologist/80783#:~:text=%2D%2D%20The%20
Outcome,46.1%25%20in%20the%20control%20patients.

142 https://www.ornish.com/undo-it/

143 https://www.healthline.com/nutrition/ornish-diet-review

144 https://www.medpagetoday.com/opinion/skepti-
cal-cardiologist/80783#:~:text=%2D%2D%20The%20
Outcome,46.1%25%20in%20the%20control%20patients.

145 https://www.cdc.gov/tobacco/data_statistics/index.
htm?s_cid=osh-stu-home-nav-005

146 https://www.cdc.gov/tobacco/data_statistics/fact_sheets/
adult_data/cig_smoking/index.htm#:~:text=In%20
2020%2C%20nearly%2013%20of,with%20a%20
smoking%2Drelated%20disease.

147 https://www.in.gov/indot/safety/safe-driving-tips/

148 https://www.hgtv.com/lifestyle/clean-and-organize/
detox-your-home-pictures

149 https://www.cdc.gov/healthywater/hygiene/body/index.
html#:~:text=Many%20diseases%20and%20conditions%20
can,spread%20of%20hygiene%2Drelated%20diseases.

150 https://www.healthdirect.gov.au/personal-hygiene#:~:text=-
Good%20personal%20hygiene%20is%20one,spreading%20
diseases%20to%20other%20people.

151 https://www.ncbi.nlm.nih.gov/pmc/articles/
PMC6503789/#:~:text=Oral%20microbiome%20is%20
crucial%20to,to%20manifest%20and%20cause%20disease.

152 https://www.nature.com/articles/
s41368-022-00163-7#Sec12

153 https://www.nature.com/articles/s41368-020-0082-x

154 https://www.zendium.co.uk/mouth-health/oral-microbi-
ome/how-to-boost-good-bacteria-in-your-mouth.html

155 https://ifstudies.org/blog/
does-marriage-really-make-us-healthier-and-happier

156 https://www.webmd.com/a-to-z-guides/news/20191010/
marriage-tied-to-longer-life-span-new-data-shows

157 https://www.cdc.gov/healthypets/keeping-pets-and-peo-
ple-healthy/how.html#:~:text=There%20are%20many%20
health%20benefits,depression%20by%20giving%20us%20
companionship.

158 https://oregoncounseling.com/article/how-hobbies-bene-fit-our-mental-health/#:~:text=Having%20a%20hobby%20can%20be,work%20performance%2C%20and%20increased%20happiness.

159 Sonners, J. (2020). Oxygen Under Pressure: Using Hyperbaric Oxygen to Restore Health, Reduce Inflammation, Reverse Aging and Revolutionize Health Care. Independently Published

160 Harch, P. (2016). The Oxygen Revolution, Third Edition: Hyperbaric Oxygen Therapy (HBOT): The Definitive Treatment of Traumatic Brain Injury (TBI) & other Disorders. Hatherleigh Press

161 https://www.princetonih.com/hyperbaric-oxygen-therapy?hsLang=en

162 https://www.insidernj.com/press-release/hyperbaric-oxy-gen-therapy-comes-to-princeton-integrative-health/

163 https://ftw.usatoday.com/2015/12/steve-weatherford-ex-plains-why-nfl-players-often-sleep-in-hyperbaric-chambers

164 https://lebronwire.usatoday.com/2019/01/11/lebron-james-takes-recovery-seriously-by-sleeping-in-oxy-gen-chamber/

165 https://www.sciencedirect.com/science/article/pii/S2214647416300381#:~:text=Photobiomodulation%20(PBM)%20describes%20the%20use,is%20at%20risk%20of%20dying.

166 https://www.ncbi.nlm.nih.gov/pmc/articles/PMC5505738/

167 https://www.news-medical.net/health/Infrared-Therapy-Health-Benefits-and-Risks.aspx

168 https://www.ncbi.nlm.nih.gov/pmc/articles/PMC4126803/

169 https://www.ncbi.nlm.nih.gov/pmc/articles/PMC5844808/

170 https://www.news-medical.net/health/Infrared-Therapy-Health-Benefits-and-Risks.aspx#:~:text=Infrared%20therapy%20has%20many%20roles,and%20lowering%20of%20blood%20pressure.

171 https://www.verywellhealth.com/what-is-chelation-90006#toc-history

172 https://www.mayoclinic.org/diseases-conditions/heart-disease/expert-answers/chelation-therapy/faq-20157449

173 McLeod, S. A. (2020, Dec 29). Maslow's hierarchy of needs. Simply Psychology. www.simplypsychology.org/maslow.html

174 https://www.lexico.com/definition/contribution

175 https://www.legacyproject.org/guides/whatislegacy.html

176 https://labs.selfdecode.com/blog/homa-ir/

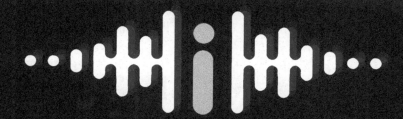

AMPLIFLUENCE
AMPLIFY YOUR INFLUENCE

You're the Expert, but are you struggling to Monetize your Authority?

Amplify Your Influence in 3 Sessions

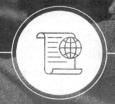

Speak Your Message

Publish Your Message

Convert Your Message

Authors and Speakers often find themselves struggling to build a strategy that actually makes them money.

Check Out All Of Our 'Live' Tour Stops

amplifluence.com

SCAN FOR TOUR INFO

More Books From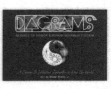

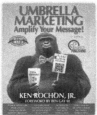 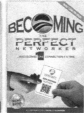 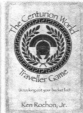 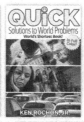

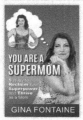 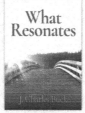 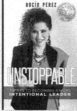 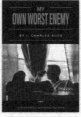 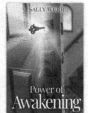

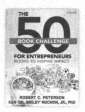 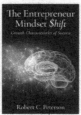 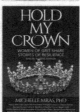 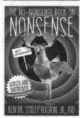 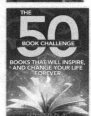

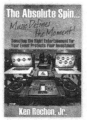 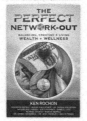 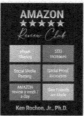 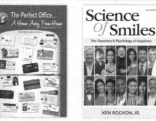

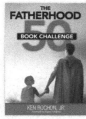 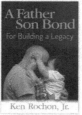 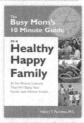 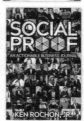 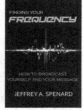

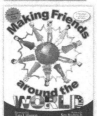 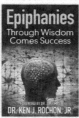 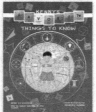 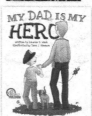 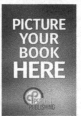

www.PerfectPublishing.com